THE
DORM
ROOM
DIET

WILLIAM MORROW

An Imprint of HarperCollins*Publishers*

THE
DORM
ROOM
DIET

REVISED & UPDATED

The 10-Step Program for Creating a Healthy
Lifestyle Plan That Really Works

FOREWORD BY Mehmet Oz, M.D.

DAPHNE OZ

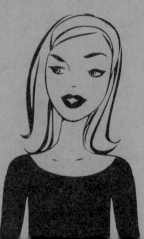

This book is designed to provide accurate and authoritative information regarding the subject matter covered. It is not intended as a substitute for medical advice from a qualified physician. The reader should consult his or her medical doctor, health adviser, or other competent professional before adopting any of the suggestions in this book or drawing inferences from them. The author and publisher specifically disclaim all responsibility for any liability, loss, or risk, personal or otherwise, that is incurred as a consequence, directly or indirectly, of the use and application of any of the contents of this book.

HarperCollins books may be purchased for educational, business, or sales promotional use. For information please write: Special Markets Departmen, HarperCollins Publishers, 10 East 53rd Street, New York, NY 10022..

FIRST WILLIAM MORROW PAPERBACK EDITION PUBLISHED 2013.

Library of Congress Cataloging-in-Publication Data

Oz, Daphne.
    Dorm room diet / Daphne Oz ; [foreword by Mehmet Oz]. — 1st ed.
        p. cm.
    Includes index.
    ISBN-13: 978-1-55704-685-7 (pbk.)
    ISBN-10: 1-55704-685-9 (pbk.)   1. College students—Nutrition.
2. College students—Health and hygiene.   3. Weight loss.   I. Title.

    RA777.3.O9 2006
    613'.0434—dc22

                                                                    2006009600

Design by Lucy Albanese.
Illustrations in Chapter 6 by Machiko.
Drawing of woman used throughout the book © 2010 Veer, a Corbis Corporation Brand.

ISBN 978-1-55704-915-5
14 15 16 17 ov/rrd 10 9 8 7 6 5 4 3

CONTENTS

Foreword, by Mehmet Oz, M.D.......vii

Acknowledgments......xiii

INTRODUCTION GET IT RIGHT, NOW.........1

STEP 1 GET INSPIRED.........13

STEP 2 GET INFORMED: THE FRESHMAN 15.........25

STEP 3 GET STARTED: HEALTHY EATING 101.........55

STEP 4 GET A GRIP: WHERE AND HOW TO
EAT RESPONSIBLY AT COLLEGE.........85

STEP 5 GET PREPARED: THE FIVE DANGER ZONES
AND HOW TO SURVIVE THEM.........107

STEP 6 GET MOVING: THE EXERCISE FACTOR.........137

STEP 7 GET YOUR VITAMINS: EVERYTHING YOU
NEED TO KNOW ABOUT SUPPLEMENTS.........175

STEP 8 GET HAPPY: A MORE RELAXED,
MORE EFFECTIVE YOU.........209

STEP 9 GET CONSCIOUS: FOOD FOR THOUGHT.........227

STEP 10 GET COOKING: RECIPES YOU CAN ENJOY.........251

References.........281

Index.........283

For my parents, Mehmet and Lisa
My sisters, Arabella and Zoe
And my brother, Oliver

FOREWORD

BY Mehmet Oz, M.D.

FOUR YEARS AGO, when my eldest daughter, Daphne, first published *The Dorm Room Diet*, I remember asking how she felt the members of her generation could take better care of themselves. "We don't need more information," she told me. "We need more relatable teachers." Her vision was to help meet this need by becoming the go-to girl for how to live healthily—and happily—for a young, busy, independent, conscious consumer.

With her first book, Daphne hoped to make the prospect of learning to eat, exercise, and supplement healthfully while living on a college campus not only possible, but fun. In this revised and expanded edition of *The Dorm Room Diet*, she takes readers one step further along the journey to health with a new focus on conscious living: seeing the relationship between food and health and personal choice on a global level. In the fight for health in America, engaging each of us to harness our consumer power for good is the next frontier. I'm a heart surgeon and a talk show host.

Today, I am fortunate to get to speak to so many proactive Americans, eager to become experts on how to best care for themselves. But I spent the better part of my career face-to-face with an open chest full of rusted arteries and rotted organs, created by a lifetime of poor health habits. My colleagues and I began to see younger and younger patients as a generation that grew up with tremendous opportunity for indulgence began to suffer from the lack of practical advice on pursuing a healthy lifestyle.

Despite their unprecedented access to information, the young men and woman on my operating table had not been able to create a lifestyle that would have preserved the health they had as children and teenagers. Sometime between the sandbox and their first apartment, these folks had missed the health boat. What Daphne realized was that college presents the perfect opportunity to forge health-promoting habits because it combines responsibility and freedom with peer-to-peer learning. But she also knew that she was up against some tough competition: namely, beer and pizza (and Xbox 360). There's a reason we hear so much about the dreaded "Freshman 15," after all.

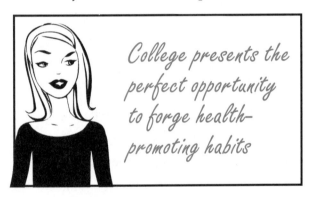

College presents the perfect opportunity to forge health-promoting habits

It starts with an extra cookie here and there, and then maybe the Sunday doughnut turns into the Sunday/Monday/twice-on-Saturday doughnut. A few more snacks, an extra scoop of soft serve, three slices of pizza instead of two. In college, studying hard (and perhaps socializing even harder) means you skip the gym and skimp on eating right. And by the time *American Idol* comes on, you'd rather flop on the couch than flip off the TV. Eventually, the only part of your body that's getting any exercise is your right thumb. (In my day, there wasn't any running involved in keg races.)

Soon, your clothes are too small and your belly is too big. And then one day—maybe it's a look in the mirror, or a picture of you wearing a bathing suit on spring break, or spotting all the buttons that have plummeted to their closet-floor graves—you realize you're built like a Monday night cafeteria special: all mush.

Without question, this is the single biggest health threat in our country: we're fat. We're a country of big portions, supersizing and deep-frying, and our clothes now have more Xs on the label than an adult video. In fact, the adolescent obesity rate has more than doubled since I was a kid, thirty years ago. Many of these people suffer from loss of self-esteem, low energy, diminishing of their intellectual prowess, an increased incidence of wrinkles, and even difficulty achieving orgasm (yes, you read right). The sad truth is that some of them will end up on my operating room table, when it can be too late to undo a lifetime of poor choices.

The time to intervene is when you're young—just as you're developing your own brand-new habits of eating, exercising, and purchasing. This is why advertisers focus intensely on fifteen- to thirty-year-olds. Whatever direction you start off in, you'll most likely stay that course for the next fifty years. Not many people change detergents in the middle of their lives. Same goes for eating and living habits.

By educating young folks, we have an advantage. Kids translate knowledge into action incredibly fast. Adults don't. If it comes in the right format and from the right source, information takes on new life for the sponge-like minds of young people, and it quickly becomes a part of their vernacular. Even better, adolescents are the viral marketers of a society. If you learn healthy habits, you'll share them with your siblings, parents, classmates, and eventually even your own kids. You are the trendsetters because you spread the awareness and create the demand. The hope is that you will use this incredible influence to help shift the health paradigm from my generation's—supermarket shelves lined with white bread and Spam—to a new reality of high-quality food at affordable prices, available to everyone.

So who is the right messenger to help you learn to make the right choices in your life and spread the word to others? Not me, not your parents, not even your teachers. Your best teachers are one another. You understand each other not only because you like the same music and movies, but you come from the same cultural cooking pot. You have similar concerns about our planet, and you're savvy about the impact our daily decisions can make. Most importantly, you share the same challenges to keeping the most precious inheritance anyone can have, your body, working in high gear—challenges such as busy schedules, fat-infused dorm food, irregular sleep patterns, and a priority list on which eating right rarely makes an appearance.

My daughter Daphne is a recent college graduate who is now navigating independent life in her first apartment and a whole new slew of challenges. But she continues to rely on the tips and tricks she developed as a college freshman when she realized how important it was to establish healthy habits that would last her a lifetime. Like you, she was worried about the difficulties of juggling healthy living with college fun. But she had a unique set of skills that let her create a manual that works, and has since struck a working balance, in school and beyond.

She has a probing, insightful mind. She has also had the advantage of a lifelong education on how to keep her body and brain honed and toned. From me she has amassed the well-researched, scientific information about healthy living. From her mother she has learned how to live on a healthy vegetarian diet. From her grandmother, a nutritional adviser, she has garnered a wealth of information about the proper use of supplements. But even with this extra boost of lifestyle education, Daphne traveled a rough road on the journey to eating and exercising right. Once she found a plan that worked for her, she put all this information together for the benefit of readers her own age, in the magazine language she honed as a writer for *ELLEgirl* magazine (so she can make the point while you enjoy the ride). And now that she has weathered a few years on her own and learned the pitfalls college and life thereafter can pose to your health, she's revised and updated the original plan to meet the needs of a new class of co-eds. In this guidebook, she shares her solutions.

I know personally that the store of knowledge she shares in this book was hard-won over many years. Daphne has gathered an impressive amount of advice and information, and she brings the message alive with news that you can use. This book provides an invaluable blueprint for you to make the crucial decisions that will become your lifestyle routines. It will teach you how to navigate the serpentine path to living well and how to make the right choices and turn them into the habits that will make you feel and look healthy, confident, and cool. Moreover, it will give you the tools you need to make your eating choices count so that they benefit you and the planet we inhabit. And it won't hurt a bit. Trust me—she knows what she's talking about.

ACKNOWLEDGMENTS

THIS BOOK WOULD not have been possible without the expert guidance and passionate enthusiasm of the Newmarket Press team, headed up by Esther Margolis, a brilliant leader and compassionate heart who believed in this book from the beginning. My editor, Theresa Burns, engineered the creation of this book. Without her innate understanding of what was needed (and her unparalleled ability to get me to write just that!), I would not have been able to hand in a single chapter. Keith Hollaman and Linda Carbone worked tirelessly to compile all of the elements and make sure that no corners were cut, whether in the production process itself or in planning for future publicity. (And Keith's own wife, Machiko, did the beautiful illustrations!) Harry Burton, publicity wizard, made sure that no refrigerator would be without its own *Dorm Room Diet* magnet. Thanks also to Heidi Sachner for her sales savvy and input of ideas throughout the process. Lucy Albanese's lively page design and Mary Schuck's cover design really brought this book to life. I am indebted to you all.

ACKNOWLEDGMENTS

I would also like to thank Joel Nash—the world's greatest personal trainer, not to mention Calvin Klein underwear model. Thanks to him, every dorm room can become the in-home gym we've all been waiting for.

My father, Dr. Mehmet Oz, deserves full credit for making sure that neither I, nor anybody else, dropped the ball. He believed in this book from its very inception and ensured that it matured into the most complete work we could compile. He led by example, and I am so grateful to have had his excellent mentorship. My mother, Lisa Oz, a creative genius, was the person responsible for such great ideas as including dorm-personalized workouts, even as she insisted that this book needed to be a total wellness manual, focusing on spiritual and emotional health, not just physical.

My grandparents Dr. Gerald Lemole and Mrs. Emily Jane Lemole were fountains of information. Without their expertise and complete patience in helping me to understand a small fraction of their knowledge, no part of this book could have been created. And my grandparents Dr. Mustafa Oz and Mrs. Suna Oz supported me through the difficult parts of the writing process. They instilled in me the work ethic to push through the tough parts of any process and always do my best.

Finally, I would like to thank the students of Dwight-Englewood School and Princeton University, who generously contributed their experiences, comments, queries, criticisms, and requests so that this book could best address its target audience.

INTRODUCTION
GET IT RIGHT, NOW

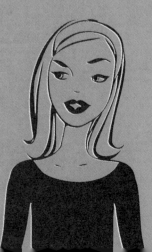

I MAGINE YOU'RE A freshman at Fat U. You pummel the alarm clock as it sounds the end of a not-so-restful night's sleep, thanks to the pizza you shared with your roommate at midnight. Groggily, you find your way to the bathroom, cautiously peer into the mirror, and find your face is a mass of dark circles, puffy eyes, and zits. You go through your face-cleaning regimen, applying harsh chemicals to your troubled skin. Because this process takes so long, you don't have time for a good breakfast, and you run out of the dorm, frazzled and starving. The fact that your belly is hanging over the pants that used to be your "fat jeans" doesn't improve matters any. "How did I get myself into this mess?!" you wonder, unwrapping a half-crushed candy bar you find at the bottom of your purse. Classes drone on, you find yourself unable to concentrate, and by lunchtime you are craving another sugar-and-carb fix. You fall asleep at the library after lunch, trudge back to the dorm, and collapse on the couch for a "power nap." You wake up four hours later, feeling more tired than before and furious because now you have to do homework rather than go to the movies with friends, as you had planned.

Now, imagine you are a freshman at Fit U. Instead of feeling groggy and slow when the alarm clock buzzes, you feel energized and alert. "Good thing I passed on that pizza last night," you think to yourself. In the bathroom, you throw some warm water on your face and are happy to see that there's not a blemish in sight and your eyes look wide and well rested. You bound back to your room and get dressed. You don't have to spend time trying on several different outfits because everything looks great, so you've got five minutes to spare: just enough time for a low-fat yogurt and a piece of fruit for breakfast. Feeling calm and rejuvenated, you practically float into class (heads turn, choirs sing, etc.) and find that time passes quickly because your brain has the proper nutrients and can concentrate on what is being taught. Lunchtime arrives and you're hungry, but not starving. You enjoy your tuna on whole wheat, and aren't even tempted by the cookies that are so conveniently placed by the checkout counter. Your afternoon class breezes by—well, as breezily as calculus can. Later, you finish your homework with enough time to run to the gym for a forty-minute cardio session. After your shower, you're ready to go to the movies with friends as you had planned. At the end of the night, you climb into bed and quickly fall into a restful sleep.

What made the difference between the Fat U student and the Fit U student? Simple: lifestyle and eating habits. While our Fat U student opted to save time by cramming down simple carbohydrates and sugar-loaded snacks, in the end she suffered because of her poor nutrition. Our Fit U student, on the other hand, began her day with a healthy meal, empowering her body to do its work effectively and establishing a cycle of restful sleep, clear skin, high energy, healthy body image, and overall satisfaction and happiness.

Okay, so maybe these examples are a little exaggerated. But figuring out how to eat healthfully on your own without your parents' guidance is one of the hardest lessons you must learn when you leave home for college. Whether you grew up in a home where healthy eating and purposeful activity were priorities or where fast food was a frequent standby and physical exercise was never on the agenda, college can pose a huge threat to anyone's jeans. If you're not careful, it is easy to lose good habits you learned at home, or reinforce bad ones.

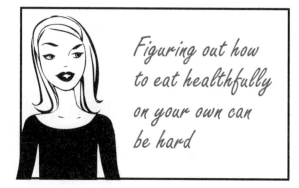

Figuring out how to eat healthfully on your own can be hard

If you find yourself on a couch in the student lounge face-to-face with a mountain of junk food wrappers, you know it's time to make some changes.

While calorie-counting programs or trendy quick-fix diets might seem like the easy way out if you want to lose weight fast, these strict regimens are not long-term solutions. For one thing, some recommend extremely unhealthy eating habits, such as consuming really high levels of protein and no fruits or veggies. For another, they are often hard to follow, especially when you're surrounded by friends who aren't watching what they eat and you live in a place that doesn't exactly cater to the health conscious. (See how long your no-carbs rule lasts when you're looking to get a late-night snack delivered and pizza is the only option.) Most importantly, fad diets throw everything out of perspective and give food more power than it should ever have. When you're in control of your eating habits, it's easy to recognize that food is there for fuel (and enjoyment). Most quick-fix plans force you to see food as the enemy because it is so often "off limits." In most cases, it's only a matter of time before you go off your diet and binge your way through several forbidden items. For all your days or weeks or months of suffering, you're right back where you started (if you're lucky). Even worse, your relationship with food is completely out of whack. Why bother with all this negative energy? Rather than torture yourself (and anyone around you) by limiting your eating to a few, select items, why not try a plan that lets you decide where, when, and what to eat? When you're in control of the "rules" of your eating, you're in control of the outcome of your eating, too.

A *diet* is simply the eating plan followed by a certain individual. But, these days, just *seeing* the word "diet" conjures up feelings of anxiety and insecurity, sending the average female into a frenzied state in which no food is safe—we're talking everything from yesterday's leftovers to your friend's half-eaten cookie. We say "going on a diet" because diets have come to represent a "going away" from normal behavior, a temporary period of self-inflicted suffering. Call me dramatic, but when we force ourselves to follow eating patterns that are often both unhealthy and inconvenient, seeing how long we can last before we crack under the strain, subjecting ourselves to the depression and fatigue that come from not having a balanced food intake, and longing for foods that are off-limits, do we actually believe that we are getting healthier? With restrictive diets, it's a race against time: do you really want to see how long you can last?

The Dorm Room Diet is nothing like the conventional diets you may have tried in the past. It offers guidelines for creating a healthy lifestyle on your own, without the daunting restrictions of a quick-fix diet. Most of us eat not only when we're hungry, but also when we're thirsty, bored, sad, or happy. This book will help you stop eating out of emotional need and put food back in its proper place, minus all the feelings of guilt and shame. On the Dorm Room Diet plan, you choose when to indulge, and you choose how much is enough. You'll be amazed by how little it takes to satisfy your cravings once nothing is "off limits." As previously forbidden items start to lose their mystique, you'll be on a path to a happier, healthier, more satisfied you.

This book will give you the tools to understand how what you put in your mouth affects the way your body functions and looks day in and day out. You'll never make decisions, at least about eating, from a place of ignorance. Clichéd as it sounds, knowledge is power. With the knowledge you gain in this book, you will have the power to take the exhilarating independence that comes with going away to college and use it to transform yourself into the healthy adult you want to be. Since you make the rules, you won't need to worry about whether that brownie is within the guidelines. The brownie is in if you say it is. Now, doesn't that sound like a piece of cake?

Think of this book as your 10-step program for achieving and maintaining your new healthy lifestyle. While you may want to consult more specialized texts if you are dealing with certain dietary restrictions or other health issues, this book will help you stay healthy—and happy—at college and beyond. Step 1 offers you some words of inspiration, and ideas for motivation, as you begin to establish your goals. Step 2 looks at the reasons college students especially—and young people in general—find it so difficult to commit to a program of healthy eating, and explains how to move beyond these obstacles. Steps 3 and 4 examine when, where, and especially *what* to eat while at school (or anytime

Think of this book as your 10-step program for achieving and maintaining your new healthy lifestyle

you're away from home), to make your mind alert and your body strong and resilient. Once you understand, for example, how simple carbs and sugars send your blood glucose levels soaring, then plummeting, propelling you into a coma-like state from which your only rescue is another sugar fix, that brownie we just talked about will seem a lot less appealing.

Unfortunately, sometimes the stress, boredom, or even happiness we experience at college can prove too overwhelming for even the most disciplined eaters. Step 5 will show you how to navigate some of the most common college danger zones in which you'll be tempted to let food have its way with you. Step 6 describes the importance of exercise and explains how to tailor a weekly workout regime around your busy schedule—even in the tiniest of dorm rooms—with the help of celebrity trainer Joel Harper. In Step 7, we'll look at how important natural remedies and supplements can be to make up for nutritional lapses, as well as to treat minor ailments. Step 8 presents practical ways to relax and rejuvenate yourself right on campus, so you can stay mentally and emotionally healthy, as well. Step 9 will help you to see how you can start demanding access to health everywhere you go by becoming a conscious eater, day in and day out. This means knowing where your food came from, how it was grown, how it got to you, and whether or not you're going to choose to support these practices—you have all the power! And finally, Step 10 will give you all sorts of fun-to-make recipes to give your eating plan variety and pizzazz. My hope is that, once you have all the information in front of you, you'll become as passionate about "living consciously" as I have and join me in spreading the word. Trust me: we'll have fun.

My dad, who is a heart surgeon, works with many adult patients who did not take good care of their bodies in their formative years. He is able to teach them how to break old eating and exercise habits and reshape their bodies, but not without a great deal of resistance. The thing is, once you've lived your life eating a doughnut for breakfast every day, a double cheeseburger for lunch, and steak and potatoes for dinner, it can be very hard to adopt a new eating pattern that includes more natural, raw foods and less processed garbage. Most of my dad's patients probably wouldn't change their ways if they weren't suffering and facing death as a direct result of their bad eating habits. The good news for us is this: we're still young. We haven't developed habits that are set in stone yet. Granted, we probably don't have the prospect of death from cardiovascular failure as incentive to change any bad habits we do have—but is that

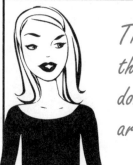

The good news for us is this: we're still young—we don't yet have habits that are set in stone

really a bad thing? It's relatively easy, and enormously important, for us to learn now the skills that will keep us healthy for the rest of our lives. By reading this far, you've already begun the process.

So you're probably wondering who I am and what gives me the credentials to write such a book? As you might have guessed, I haven't been to grad school, and there's no M.D. after my name. I'm a recent college grad who just happens to spend her free time reading up on the latest in nutritional research and the various health-promoting practices of the day. Additionally, I grew up with a father and two grandfathers who are heart surgeons, and an uncle who is a neurosurgeon. My grandma is a specialist in homeopathic remedies and complementary medicine. (Basically, she knows a lot about vitamin supplementation, natural remedies, and proper eating.) And my mom is a practicing vegetarian and reiki master. With all these health experts in my family, I grew up hearing about what I *should* be eating, what I *should* be taking for vitamins, and how I *should* be exercising to maintain ideal health. Of course, what I *should* have done is not always what I did.

Even with all that medical knowledge surrounding me, from the time

I was seven until I was seventeen I was overweight. At my heaviest, I was 5'8" and 175 pounds. I ate well, but in too large quantities, and I rarely made a concerted effort to burn off the extra calories. I'd beat myself up about being overweight, even though I had the tools to be in shape. Then I'd resort to an unhealthy diet to lose the weight that was making

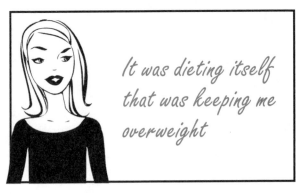

It was dieting itself that was keeping me overweight

me self-conscious. Because being on a diet added to my insecurity, when the weight didn't come off or came off too slowly, I quickly fell back into old habits and food once again became a comfort. It sounds like a psychotic seesaw, but this is often the way insecurities feed off one another. Because I hadn't made a decision to change my lifestyle, it was impossible for me to keep the weight off. It was dieting itself that was keeping me overweight.

I was only able to lose—and keep off—the 30 extra pounds I was lugging around once I stopped treating food as an emotional crutch and put it back in perspective as the fuel that it is. Once I made the rules about when to eat (basically, whenever my body truly needed refueling, with a few treats here and there), I could pretty much eat what I wanted. When I stopped feeding emotional hunger with food, I stopped having to worry about never feeling satisfied. Gradually, what I ate began to shift toward the healthier end of the spectrum. And success led to success. Once I was able to reorganize my eating life, the rest took care of itself. Six years down the road and well out of college, leading a healthy lifestyle that provides all the nutrition I need, while allowing for indulging in moderation, has become second nature to me.

I'll talk more specifically about my journey in Step 1, but the point I'm trying to make is that I know what it's like to be the "big girl." I know how much you want to do what is in your own best interest, and I know how badly you want to look and feel your best. This book—and your own commitment to success—are all you need to create a plan that works for you. Now let's take that first step.

STEP 1

GET INSPIRED

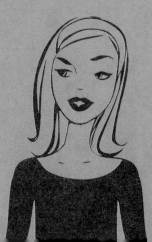

A T THIS POINT you may be thinking, "I am so sick of these self-help books telling me how easy it is to lose weight and get healthy. If it were so easy to lose weight, don't you think I would have done it already?"

Allow me to clarify: It's only easy to lose weight and become healthy once you get over the *fear* of succeeding. I'm convinced that it's not fear of failure but fear of success that's keeping you from committing your entire self to changing the lifestyle that has made you unhealthy. After all, if you are successful in establishing a healthy lifestyle (which you would be if you committed to it 100 percent), think about everything that would have to change. You'd probably have to adjust your life, perhaps in some uncomfortable ways, to accommodate the new you. For one thing, you'd have to get a whole new wardrobe. You'd focus on wanting to feed your body what it needed for you to feel and look your best, rather than sticking to the popular fad diets of the day. Friends and family might treat you differently—they might feel guilty for not wanting to change their habits. They might even resent the success you're experiencing. And after you've achieved this slimmer, healthier you, you'll have to maintain it forever—or, once again, risk looking like a failure. So, you figure, "Why rock the boat?"

The easiest way I found to overcome this fear of changing a little bit in order to get big results is to prove to yourself that you really do want things to be different. And that means finding your inspiration—the thing that motivates you not just to *think* about changing, but actually to take the steps that get you there. That's why I'm going to tell you about my life as an unhealthy child and teenager, so that I can show you all the times when I revealed just how unhappy I was and how badly I wanted to make a change.

In preschool, I was the largest kid in the class, standing at least a head above the next tallest child. Being taller than everyone else didn't really bother me, but being bigger than every other child did. On one occasion, my mother and I were in an elevator and another passenger, thinking it odd that a five-year-old (little did he know I was only two at the time) could not form full sentences, asked my mother how she was getting along raising a "slow" child. Clearly not the most tactful question, but it does illustrate how large I was for my age, a fact that would stick with me for seventeen years. Of course, the phase of being taller than everyone ended, especially once the boys hit puberty and sprouted another two or three feet. But the "bigger" portion of the equation stayed in place.

Now, don't think I stayed heavy for any lack of incentive. Though I was rarely assaulted with fat-kid jokes, there were more subtle slights that proved just as hurtful. For instance, I was never the last person picked when choosing up teams in gym class, probably because my size proved helpful in annihilating smaller, opposing players. But it earned me the affectionate nickname Bulldozer. As anyone who has ever been the target of verbal abuse or criticism will understand, once you've heard something said about you enough times, you grow to believe it. At no point in my childhood did I think of myself as graceful or feminine; bulldozers are neither of these things.

As an adolescent, I believed that looks were far more important than health. I didn't really give much thought to the health problems my weight posed, though there were plenty of these, as I would later find out. I cared about how my classmates and my family, and society in general, perceived me. All the magazines and movies told me that thin was pretty, as did the stores around my house that only carried pants through size 8. Being a size 12 meant I was undesirable, unattractive.

I would become depressed whenever I saw pictures of myself from family vacations. I found it extremely difficult to take a "good" photo, and demanded to be allowed to destroy all the pictures in which I looked like a "beached whale." Whether I actually looked as awful as I thought, I'll never know; I have few pieces of photographic evidence left from those years. I seesawed between denying to myself that I was overweight, which meant I did not have to monitor what I ate and when I exercised, and accepting that I was overweight and was doomed to stay that way, which meant that I didn't have to make any effort to change.

My father knew the dangers of being overweight and would constantly urge me to be more active and to eat more healthfully. My mother, a vegetarian, never cooked us meats, so I didn't have to worry about fatty steaks or hamburgers. (Refined carbohydrates, such as pasta and bread, and starchy vegetables, like potatoes, are the equivalent for vegetarians.) My diet, which incorporated mainly healthy foods, did not incorporate moderation. I would consume huge portions of whatever it was I was eating. Also, because my mother rarely bought chips, candy, or soda, in an effort to keep her family fit and healthy, the temptations to consume these foods once I was out of the house was overwhelming.

Well, high school rolled around and so did I. I was overweight and unhappy. I had long, thick, dark hair that sort of hung in my face, very Cousin Itt-esque, and, I would slouch around campus wondering why God was smiting me. Denying that my eating was part of the problem allowed me to avoid having to change my lifestyle. While I frequented the gym more often once I got to high school, I would consume any calories that I burned off, and then some. If I went to the gym and burned, say, 300 calories, that number would seem to grow in my head as the day went on. By the time I was scarfing down two slices of pizza for dinner, I'd convinced myself that I had burned off 1,000 calories earlier, and I was still way ahead of the game. Better still was tennis, basketball, or lacrosse practice, during which I had no idea how many calories I used up and could fabricate a number as high as I needed to justify the amount of food I consumed.

Actually, the sports field was the place where I struggled most as a result of my weight. My coaches recognized my skill at sports and put me on the varsity team, only to find that my weight limited my endurance and induced chronic ankle sprains and knee injuries. As a result of the extra burden my weight placed on my joints, I spent most of my athletic career on the bench.

The classroom posed its own problems. Though my overall grades were good, snacking on junk foods I could get at the cafeteria or school co-op left me chronically tired and cranky, making it difficult to concentrate on

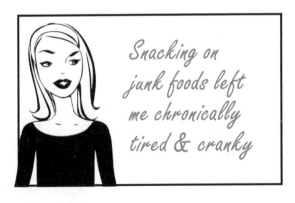

Snacking on junk foods left me chronically tired & cranky

what was being taught. I found out later that my diet of simple carbs (which are basically just sugars) contributed to my inability to focus by making me jittery and hungry all the time. These foods don't have enough fiber or fat to keep you full for very long. If you're always hungry and thinking about your next sugar-and-carb fix, of course you're going to be distracted.

Part of the reason I never felt any urgency to lose weight, despite my inability to perform at optimum levels in any arena, was that, growing up in a large family, I had learned how to attract attention and be heard. Thus, I always had a good, supportive group of friends who made me secure in my surroundings, even though I felt uncomfortable in my own skin. Also, my tight-knit family gave me unconditional love, which kept me from feeling constantly depressed about the way I looked. Other than my parents' frequent suggestion that I start eating more healthfully and becoming more active, my need to change was never outwardly affirmed. If no one else minded me being fat, why should I?

The beginning of senior year came and I found myself thinking, "Wow, I've made it through high school as one of the 'fat kids' and still managed to get everything I wanted and expected out of high school." I had taken all the honors classes; I was applying to a top college; I had plenty of friends; I had had boyfriends. Yet, the more I thought about how "content" I was with my high school experience, the more I realized how much I relied on outward affirmation to assure myself that I was happy, especially with the way I looked. What happened to liking myself? Was I supposed to settle for a mediocre me?

The time came to create the "senior page" in our yearbook: all graduating students decorate a page to commemorate themselves and their experience in high school. Usually, the page consists of a few pictures and some words saying thanks to those who made our time at school worthwhile. Because I hated the way I looked, I only picked pictures of myself as a little child. This was supposed to be a page of me in high school and I was only comfortable showing pictures of myself as I no longer was: a newborn in her parents' arms, a naked three-year-old on a Florida beach, a four-year-old in a dress-up crown. I was ashamed of what I had become. I did not want people to remember me in my current state. And yet, what was I doing about it?

It took this blatant display of self-consciousness to burst the bubble I had been living in for more than a decade. I knew it was time to forge a body that I could be proud of and that wouldn't limit me from doing all I am capable of achieving. I didn't want to be the benched varsity player, metaphorically or literally. I wanted to be the starting playmaker. Finally, I proved to myself that it didn't matter what anyone else thought. *I* wanted to make a change.

At just about the same time that I had to turn in my senior page for the yearbook, I began doing some research for a school project on teenage eating habits. I looked into the various government-recommended guidelines for teenage eating, and how well we, as a nation, followed them. Our generation is surprisingly out of sync with what we should be eating, according to experts in the field. As consumers, we fund fast food franchises that, though they began as small burger chains, are now billion-dollar industries. Even more impressive to me than the success of these companies is the impact consumers have on the direction of their growth. For instance, the introduction of various salad options at many of these establishments is a direct result of consumers demanding healthier choices on the menu. That got me thinking: What if my peers, a huge portion of the spending population and the target audience of nearly every ad company, learned about other ways to stay healthy besides living on rabbit food? And then demanded access to health on a regular basis. Just think of the difference that could make, not only in fast food chains and supermarkets, but in schools, in government programs, in city planning, in nearly every facet of life.

As I read more and more of the information doctors, researchers, and dietitians offered on what we should be eating to lead the healthiest lives possible, I noticed something else: it was tedious stuff. And, while I was greatly expanding my knowledge of the subject, it was hard work finding all the information I wanted. As a teenager, I didn't want to read long-winded documents written by extremists from my parents' generation about how we need to "cut out all refined sugars and flour." Rather than spending hours searching through a medical dictionary, I wanted clear, concise facts, carefully selected by experts so that I was only getting the information that pertained directly to my life and that suited my lifestyle. And I didn't just want to learn about eating. I also wanted information on how to exercise properly and efficiently to meet my goals. But I could not find that information in a reader-friendly format, in any of the sources I was looking through.

My friends, who knew that I was on a quest to learn as much as I could about what I should be eating, not only for my school project, but also to lose weight and be healthy myself, started coming to me with questions. "What should I eat before a big game?" "I have a test tomorrow; what foods will help fuel my brain?" I realized that I was not the only one interested in this stuff: my peers wanted to know how to get and stay healthy, too. They just couldn't figure out how to do it. I decided to put together a book so that anyone who wanted the information could get it easily.

But there still remained the issue of my losing weight. I had all the incentive I needed, even the information on what foods to eat and what exercises I should be doing, collected from a top trainer, to burn fat most efficiently while building muscle. The final turning point came when I was accepted to college. I realized that this represented an entirely new stage in my life. I would be meeting new people, living away from my family and old friends, and adjusting to a completely new environment. This was my big chance to finally start "walking the talk." If I didn't seize the opportunity to change now, when would I? So I began the process of revolutionizing my lifestyle. And I haven't looked back since.

Don't get me wrong; this was not an easy transition. There are days when it would be infinitely more desirable just to stay in bed, rather than do the cardio routine I committed myself to four times a week. The sheets are so soft, the pillow so inviting! But the stakes really are high. You just have to pinch yourself in the gut, get your lazy self out of bed, and know that what you are doing is making you healthier and more functional for the rest of your life. Going through the relative pain of working out makes eating that second helping of ice cream less fun, because you know the kind of effort that went in to working off the first scoop.

Creating a healthy lifestyle for yourself is not about deprivation. It's about *consciousness*. Whenever the temptation to eat junk food arises, I have to consciously make the decision to indulge or not. If I choose to eat something "bad," I don't feel the need to eat massive quantities; I can be satisfied with a few bites. I am still in the process of making myself as healthy as possible, and always will be. But I've realized that in order to make my commitment to a healthy lifestyle last, I need to be flexible. I don't graze mindlessly, but I also never let myself feel deprived—indulgence in moderation is the key to success. By creating a habit of exercising daily

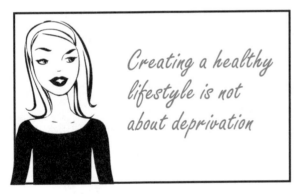

Creating a healthy lifestyle is not about deprivation

(though not necessarily in a gym) and always being conscious of what I am eating, I am on my way to a healthier me. And you will be, too.

By the time I arrived at college in my freshman year, I had lost a total of 10 pounds. And I took off another 10 pounds in my first three months at school. As you probably know, losing weight in your freshman year is no small feat. I got lucky because my roommate happened to be a rower on the crew team, so health and fitness were top priorities for her and her habits reinforced my own fitness goals. But that is not always the case. At college, there are so many new stresses to deal with, new opportunities to eat unhealthily, and new people to influence your eating and exercising habits negatively. Thankfully, for each of these challenges, there is a positive choice available to you.

By developing my own eating alternatives (such as chocolate-dipped strawberries instead of a candy bar, sparkling water and juice rather than soda, even sorbet instead of ice cream) and removing myself from places of temptation (like the snack table at parties), I was able to navigate my freshman year in a healthy way. I learned, through trial and error, what I could get away with (ice cream once a week) and what I couldn't (ice cream every day). And, on those occasions when I chose to indulge, I learned how to organize my day so that I could burn some of those calories off at the gym and still have time to relax with friends, get enough sleep, and finish my homework. If you'll let me, I would like to share this knowledge with you.

Going to college helped me get myself healthy, but only because I had the *inspiration* (all those silly baby pictures!) and the *information* (all the knowledge I picked up during my research and from my family of doctors). College proved to be my *motivation*, the catalyst that led to my lifestyle overhaul, because it marked the onset of my life as an adult. I did not want that life to mirror what my teenage years had been: a time of dishonesty and dissatisfaction with myself. Once I had the *inspiration, information*, and *motivation* I needed, I was finally able to make a *transformation*, the lifestyle change that marked the end of my willingness to settle for a second-rate me.

As a first step in your own transformation, write out the answers to the following questions. You may even want to make photocopies of this page to paste around your dorm in places where you'll be sure to notice them.

1. **WHAT IS THE PROOF THAT YOU ARE READY TO MAKE A LIFESTYLE CHANGE?** List one or two things that make you feel insecure, like trying clothes on or going to the beach. If you've had any sort of epiphany, as I did making my senior page, list that.

2. **HOW CAN YOU BE SURE THAT YOU ARE READY TO MAKE THE COMMITMENT TO A HEALTHIER YOU?** List the reasons why now is the time for change, as opposed to any other time that you've tried to make a transformation.

3. **WHAT IS SOMETHING YOU HAVE BEEN SUCCESSFUL AT BEFORE?** Maybe you got accepted to an internship you really wanted, or got an A on that impossible final exam. Write down some successes that you are proud of.

4. **HOW WERE YOU ABLE TO OVERCOME ANY OBSTACLES THAT STOOD IN THE WAY OF YOUR BEING SUCCESSFUL?** Your answer to this question is really important, as you may be able to use the same techniques to push yourself past the challenges that will present themselves as you try to get healthy.

5. **WHAT IS YOUR FIRST SHORT-TERM GOAL TO BECOMING A HEALTHIER PERSON?** When I say "short-term," I mean something you can accomplish in the next week. You can decide to stop eating two hours before bed, or start drinking a glass of water before every meal, or go to the gym three times a week. Make it a simple goal that you're sure you can accomplish and use to give yourself a boost of confidence.

STEP 2

GET INFORMED

The Freshman 15

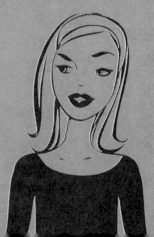

M ENTION THE WORDS *Freshman 15* to any red-blooded female and watch a shudder run down her spine. Thankfully, the dread this popular catchphrase elicits is only partly justified. On average, only about 6 percent of American college sophomores report gaining 15 or more pounds during their freshman year (although 50 percent of an average freshman class can expect to gain between 2 and 5 pounds). But the *idea* that tremendous weight gain is unavoidable as a freshman has a powerful hold on many young women.

This assumption has multiple effects, ranging from obsessive dieting to complete abandon. Bethany, a high school senior of average height and build, told me she planned to lose 20 pounds before entering college to compensate for the 15 she was *sure* to gain within the first few months. Another senior I spoke with, Carla, said that she felt completely comfortable with her body image. Once in college, she would simply continue eating what she ate all through high school, and did not expect to experience any shift in weight.

As a seasoned woman—of nineteen—I felt it was my place to tell each of these naïves that such plans were easier made than followed. My purpose was not to crush Bethany's hope to lose weight, or Carla's faith in her good habits. But college is hugely different from home, and this change in environment can (and probably will) have a profound effect on your eating habits, in ways you may never have imagined. Bethany did, in fact, lose 10 pounds before starting her freshman year. While it was not as much as she'd wanted, her new roommate was a health nut and helped Bethany keep on track, so she gained only 4 pounds her entire freshman year—a net loss of 6 pounds. Carla, on the other hand, discovered how much her parents' strict eating rules (no TV watching while eating, no dessert except on weekends) had constrained her diet while at home. To her great surprise, without her parents' restrictions, she gained 13 pounds in her first semester.

It's difficult to predict what challenges college has in store for your health. But that doesn't mean you have to go crazy worrying about it in advance. Armed with the right information, you can be aware of how and why students tend to gain weight and start establishing good habits as soon as you unpack your bags.

A college campus is completely different from the home you lived in for the first eighteen years of your life. You eat on your own or with friends; you have autonomy over what goes into your mouth; you eat at irregular times and often based on convenience and budget, rather than on hunger or nutrition. Food helps you socialize, kill boredom, and cope with stress, not to mention replace the comforts of home—the home cooking as well as the support of family. Eating may or may not have filled all these roles while you were still at home. How you and your family viewed food while you were growing up will have an enormous impact on how well you adjust to eating in your new college setting. So let's stop and create a portrait of how family life influenced the way you feel about food now, and how you'll feel about it when you're living on your own.

YOUR FAMILY EATING PORTRAIT

Answer the following questions about how you and your family ate while you were living at home. They'll help you get an idea of how the choices you made and the rules you followed (or didn't follow) at home helped to create the eating habits you brought to school with you.

1. **HOW MANY MEALS DID YOU EAT PER DAY?**

2. **HOW REGULAR WERE THESE MEALS—DID THEY FALL WITHIN ONE HOUR OF THE SAME TIME EACH DAY?**

3. **DID YOU EAT SNACKS?** If so, how many daily? Were these snacks generally prepackaged or freshly prepared (nuts, fruits, veggies, and yogurt count as freshly prepared)?

4. **HOW MANY MEALS, PER DAY, DID YOU EAT WITH ANOTHER PERSON?** How often did you eat sitting down with your entire family?

5. **WOULD YOU SAY THAT YOUR MEALS WERE "RUSHED" OR "RELAXED"?** Did you take time to enjoy your food?

6. **DID YOU REGULARLY EAT WHILE WATCHING TV, TALKING ONLINE OR ON THE PHONE, OR OTHERWISE DISTRACTED?**

7. **HOW MANY MEALS, PER DAY, DID YOU PREPARE FOR YOURSELF?**

8. DID YOU HELP PLAN MEALS OR DID YOU EAT WHAT WAS PUT ON THE TABLE?

9. HOW OFTEN (THAT IS, HOW MANY MEALS PER WEEK) DID YOU EAT IN A RESTAURANT OR ORDER TAKEOUT?

10. DID YOU PREFER HOME-COOKED MEALS OR SOMETHING MADE OUTSIDE THE HOME?

11. HOW HEALTHFULLY, ON A SCALE OF 1 TO 10, 10 BEING THE MOST HEALTHY, DO YOU THINK YOUR FAMILY EATS? Your close friends?

12. ON THE SAME SCALE OF 1 TO 10, HOW HEALTHFULLY DO YOU THINK YOU EAT NOW?

13. WOULD YOU SAY THAT YOU ARE AWARE OF WHAT YOU *SHOULD* BE EATING, IN TERMS OF HOW MANY SERVINGS OF FRUITS, VEGGIES, CARBOHYDRATES, PROTEINS, AND FATS YOU SHOULD BE GETTING DAILY? If yes, how successful, on a scale of 1 to 5 (5 being very successful), are you at following these guidelines?

14. IF YOU ANSWERED "YES" TO QUESTION 13, PLEASE LIST THE SOURCE OF YOUR INFORMATION (PARENTS, INTERNET, TEACHER, AND SO ON).

15. WHAT IS THE SINGLE BIGGEST OBSTACLE YOU FACE TO EATING HEALTHFULLY?

What did you learn about your family's eating habits and attitudes from answering these questions? Maybe you never realized how much, or how little, control you had over what, when, and how you ate. If your parents were very hands-off about scheduling and eating meals, you may have made a lot of your own food decisions, which may have left you overweight and unhealthy. On the other end of the spectrum, if your parents made all the choices for you, leaving you no opportunity to develop self-discipline, it may have had the same result.

What's important at this point is to recognize how the habits you learned at home affect your health and to begin making changes. For instance, if you learned that at home you usually ate while doing something else—talking on the phone or watching TV, for instance—understand that being preoccupied while you eat keeps you from (a) enjoying the food you're eating and (b) being aware of when you've had enough, which can lead to overeating. Or maybe you saw that having to prepare meals for your little sister made you more health conscious, because you felt responsible for making sure she ate well. Whatever you realized about yourself by creating this brief portrait, now it's up to you to take this information and use it to help yourself. The good news is that, even if your family life left you with less-than-perfect eating habits, college provides a fresh start and is a great place to take control of your health.

Here are three easy steps you can follow to start eating healthfully right away:

1. DRINK A GLASS (OR TWO) OF WATER BEFORE YOU EAT ANY MEAL.

2. **TRY NOT TO EAT WHEN YOU ARE DISTRACTED (WATCHING TV, USING THE INTERNET, AT PARTIES).** The food you are most likely to eat in these settings is probably processed junk anyway and you'll end up gorging on snacks that won't keep you full. Your goal is to be *conscious* of what you eat at all times, so that you actually get to enjoy your food.

3. **TRY NOT TO EAT LESS THAN TWO HOURS BEFORE BED.** You'll guarantee yourself a better night's sleep. When you eat just before going to bed, the digestive process is still in high gear, making you sleep less deeply, not to mention that you don't give yourself any time to burn off these calories.

SUPERSIZE THIS!

Family habits can't be the only reason so many of us are worried about our health. Is it any wonder that 65 percent of all Americans are currently overweight, given the contents of the Standard American Diet (sometimes aptly referred to as SAD)? Unfortunately for us, the SAD is chock full of fats and processed foods, and low in complex carbohydrates and fiber—in other words, it is the perfect regimen to put us at risk for cancer, heart disease, stroke, and a litany of other ailments. We subsist primarily on processed, refined carbohydrates (read cookies, pretzels, French fries), since these are the cheapest, least perishable, and fastest kinds of food to grab. What's truly *sad* about the SAD is that, even though we have no shortage of fresh fruits and vegetables, lean, high-value protein, and low-fat dairy items in our rich country, we continue to live on the most nutritionally bankrupt products. In this way we actually *give* ourselves diseases.

So, why do we make these choices? Some say it's because processed foods taste better than fresh ones. Now, even I can't deny how delectable those first couple of potato chips are. But once you've swallowed and that salty taste sensation is gone, all that remains are a few hundred extra calories in your belly, artery-clogging fat seeping into your bloodstream, and greasy fingers.

But what about cost? Most college students are on a pretty tight budget. Well, processed foods do tend to be less expensive than most fresh foods. In part, they're that cheap because the U.S. government subsidizes the producers of corn and wheat, the main ingredients in those packaged snacks, which helps keep crop prices low. In addition, lean meats and fish, as well as fresh fruits and vegetables, are highly perishable items, and there's a cost involved in delivering them unsullied to your table or cafeteria tray. But the fast food burger does not necessarily need to be less expensive than the garden salad. Fresh, wholesome foods are not intrinsically more expensive to produce. Underlying most of the food price disparity in America is the fact that we, the consumers, have voted with our forks and told our government and food suppliers that all we want is cheap, convenient processed junk. Therefore, our government subsidizes crops that provide these food-like products (corn, soybeans, and wheat) so that they become very cheap to purchase and the most profitable for farmers to grow. I'll talk more about how our food supply has come to be dominated by a few select crops in chapter 9. For now, suffice it to say that yes, it is currently more expensive to eat healthy foods. (You'll see this price gap most starkly when you and your roommates decide to order dinner: one large pizza feeds three people for $12, while sushi for three can cost more than $40.) But the good news is that, with educated consumers like you, who know the power of your wallet and your mouth, this will not always have to be the case. Everyone can have access to health once we make healthy food affordable. In the meantime, start looking at your health as an investment: the cost of dealing with poor eating habits when you get older—future medical bills for everything from heart disease, to diabetes, to a shrink for your "fat issues"—easily outweighs the relatively small price difference you pay today. So cough up the extra cash and choose something healthy.

COUCH—AND CHAIR—POTATOES

Historically, Americans have often chosen to eat according to the three Cs: consistency, cheapness, and convenience. This is how fast food chains came to be so prevalent. But why, if Americans have been eating unhealthy foods for years, is obesity, and in particular teen obesity, only recently being recognized as an "epidemic"? Dr. Keith-Thomas Ayoob, associate clinical professor of pediatrics at the Albert Einstein College of Medicine in New York City, does not attribute this phenomenon to any significant increase in the amount of food consumed by American teenagers over previous decades. In other words, it's not the result of a recent spike in gluttony. Rather, Ayoob blames the three Ns—Nintendo, Netscape, and Nickelodeon—for the surge in young people's sedentary behavior in recent years. Because the number of hours in a day has not changed, the more time we spend sitting on our butts, the less time we have to devote to burning calories through physical activity. How could our overeating not catch up with us?

Think about it. How many ways can you get in touch with someone in the next room? I'll bet you thought of phone, e-mail, AIM, yelling, maybe even pounding on the wall. At what point did physically walking into the next room occur as an option? Technology has so streamlined our lives that physical exertion is largely unnecessary. (Apparently, walking from the computer chair to the couch isn't really cutting it for the forty-five-minute, thrice-weekly exercise schedule doctors recommend for young adults.) Researcher Lisa Sutherland of the University of North Carolina at Chapel Hill analyzed federal data on the diet, weight, and physical activity of teens, aged twelve to nineteen. From 1980 to 2000, there was a 1 percent increase in calories eaten and a 10 percent rise in obesity. The reason? Physical activity dropped 13 percent.

For many teens today, it's likely a combination of eating too much—the average teen consumes about 2,290 calories per day, but most teenaged females only need 1,300 to 1,800 calories daily—and not exercising that really packs on the pounds. You need to burn off as many calories as you take in in order to avoid weight gain. Depending on how well you were able to balance the energy input/energy output equation as a teenager living at home, you will need to make adjustments once you get to college. And you'll need to do this while dealing with the wholly new experience that is campus life.

COLLEGE PITFALLS

If you let it, college can prove to be a disastrous time for your health. Why? Before college, you are still considered a child. You are viewed as an extension of your parents or guardians. After college, however, you are expected to get a job, go on to higher education, and perhaps settle down and start a family of your own. You've become your own person, independent of your parents. The time you spend in college is when you find yourself, clichéd as that might sound. College life presents you with a slew of new challenges and pressures, all of which teach you how to handle life as an adult. But, if you don't see them coming, they could send you hurtling into a dependency on, among other things, food.

Before I left home for my freshman year at Princeton University, my parents let me know that even though I was attending a rigorous school I would not be allowed to get away with poor performance. Introducing pressure #1: grades. On some level, everyone views grades as a judgment of their personal worth: How good is my work? How good am I? To this internalized valuing of grades add the fact that you are living 24/7 with hundreds, if not thousands, of your peers, all struggling to get the same grades you want, all adding to your stress.

Unfortunately, goading you to do your best in school is not the only kind of pressure these peers will exert on you. Feeling as if you have to fit in with the crowd doesn't end when you graduate from high school; many college students still find it difficult to resist doing what (it seems) everyone else around them is doing, even when they know it's a bad idea. This can apply to anything from drinking six strawberry daiquiris at an off-campus party, to eating the kind of stuff you'd never have put in your body before you got to school. Standing up to this kind of groupthink can be very difficult, but I promise you it can be done and you won't find yourself friendless.

For instance, a woman in my dorm, Lydia, told me her roommates like to wrap up long nights of studying with a trip to the university store for a pint of gourmet ice cream—each. Unfortunately, long nights are fairly common in college, so she was eating ice cream at least three times a week after midnight. Because the event had become a tradition, she felt awkward saying that she didn't want to partake. Lydia knew she wasn't eating because she was hungry; it was a way to socialize and she didn't want to feel like a party pooper. She dealt with the issue by getting a low-fat frozen yogurt or a frozen fruit bar instead of ice cream; this way she could still be with her friends and enjoy their company without all the extra calories. They teased her the first time, of course, but after a few trips many of them were choosing the healthier option, too. They didn't abandon their tradition; they just adjusted it for the better.

Most first-year college students are also subjected to the stress of having to live in the same room with a complete stranger. You have none of your own space, no privacy, no previous bond of friendship, no escape from the constant scrutiny of someone you don't even know. You might find yourself paired with a nocturnal vampire who simply refuses to do her work during the day, but who is up writing papers at 3 a.m. beneath the soothing glow of fluorescent lightbulbs. Add to this stress the fact that you are away from home for an extended period, possibly for the first time in your life. Often, it seems that [insert favorite junk food] is the only cure for homesickness. . . . If only baby carrots did the trick! Thankfully, as you make more friends and get accustomed to your new surroundings, homesickness diminishes. Heck, you may even grow fond of your roomie eventually; most people do. And, in the meantime, you'll get to practice your negotiating skills and ability to compromise.

As if roommates, homesickness, courseloads, and the stress of fitting in were not enough to deal with, college cafeterias offer a huge variety of processed carbohydrates for you to load up on, especially if you find yourself grabbing food on the go. A bagel with cream cheese is one of the most common breakfast fallbacks; a box of some sweetened, refined grain cereal is another. Both are loaded with refined flour, which turns straight into sugar a few minutes after you eat it, leaving you famished within two hours and sitting on a whole bunch of empty calories.

The communal dining experience on campus also means you are constantly eating in the company of others, which introduces a new pressure, especially for young women: eat less than everyone around you. No one wants to look like a pig who can't get food onto her fork fast enough, so girls will often, subconsciously or not, start comparing how and what they eat to the girls around them. This can sometimes lead to a subliminal, or overt, competition over who eats what and how much. Though you may have eaten communally in your high school cafeteria, you did not eat all your meals surrounded by peers. You were able to make at least some of your dining decisions in the comfort of your own home. At college, all these choices are made very public.

If you think about it, the girls around you are all under the same pressures you are to keep up with work and friends and family; sooner or later, the stress gets to everybody. Just like you, they also have the media cramming the idea that "Super thin is in" down their throats, and frustration can set in when they find themselves unable to fulfill their supermodel wannabe dream. It can create a lot of anxiety when you feel that you constantly need to compete with everyone around you—not just in terms of how thin you are, but also for a place on an athletic team, for academic standing in class, within a group of friends, or even over a certain boy. In extreme cases, these pressures can lead to an eating disorder.

HOW TO RECOGNIZE AN EATING DISORDER

Your body image—your perception of your own body and the way that you convey this vision to yourself and others—can have a huge impact on both your physical and emotional health. The inability to perceive your body in a good light can lead to lowered self-esteem and depression. People with extremely poor body images are considered to be at risk for several types of eating disorders, the most common being anorexia nervosa and bulimia.

Conservative estimates show that after puberty, 5 to 10 percent of American women today are living with some form of eating disorder. Attempting to use a diet to control your weight is one thing. Engaging in hazardous emotional eating—eating for a reason other than hunger in a way

> *5 to 10 percent of American women today are living with some form of eating disorder*

that is actually harmful to you—is potentially lethal and should be reported to a professional immediately. Please don't take chances with this sort of health hazard. Anorexics starve themselves in order to fulfill a desire to be thin. When life gets out of control, anorexics often feel that their weight is the one thing they can take charge of. Their methods of weight loss vary, but the end result, without intervention, is the same: the disease takes over and the victims are no longer in control of their diet. They never see themselves as being thin enough and may diet to fatally low weights unless they receive medical help. Hospitalization may be necessary, and psychological counseling is almost always needed to recover from the disease.

Bulimics, like anorexics, suffer from an eating disorder. The primary difference is that bulimia involves bingeing (consuming huge amounts of food) followed by purging (eliminating the foods they've just eaten), rather than starvation. Bulimics may resort to vomiting or taking laxatives in order to keep from gaining weight. Again, sufferers of this disorder want to control their weight, but things often get out of hand when individuals use gorging followed by purging as a means of handling their emotions. In the end, the disease controls them.

A distorted body image that fuels a desire to lose weight may occur to a lesser degree in people without an eating disorder, leading to unhealthy weight loss or weight gain. "Yo-yo dieting" is a term used to describe severe dieting followed by periods of nondieting when any weight that was lost is gained back, plus some. The individual then goes back into diet mode to lose the regained weight, only to go off the diet later and gain back more weight. This process is extremely debilitating, both physically and emotionally. If you are obsessed with food and are constantly depriving yourself of the foods you love, this feeling of deprivation can make you feel depressed and angry. The quickest, most accessible way to numb this pain, at least superficially, is through food. When dieting becomes necessary again, yo-yo dieters frequently choose an extreme, restrictive diet plan so that overeating or cheating again becomes unavoidable, and the vicious cycle continues. The only true solution is to seek a professional's guidance to help initiate the healing process of separating food and emotion and putting each back in its rightful place.

A WORD ON EMOTIONAL EATING

Anorexia, bulimia, and yo-yo dieting are all extreme forms of what experts call emotional eating. Emotional eating means that food is being used for something other than its intended purpose, as fuel for the body. Anorexics typically use food as a way to feel powerful in a world in which they feel weak and impotent. Bulimics typically try to control their food intake, fail when they binge, and then punish themselves through forced purging of food. Yo-yo dieters fall victim to emotional eating in another way: it becomes the primary saboteur of all the diets they try.

College life can create the type of anxiety that emotional eating soothes, simply because there is such an onslaught of new experiences, people, and rituals to figure out and get used to. Nobody gets it all right. Whether it's bad grades, bad friends, bad habits, or even bad luck, college life presents a multitude of ways for you to go off course. When everything else in your life seems like a mess, food is something you choose for yourself. It can seem like you need food to help you socialize or to cope with stress or homesickness. Maybe you really are just craving a chocolate fix. Or maybe it has more to do with the crappy day you've been having, and the need for comfort, than any actual physical need.

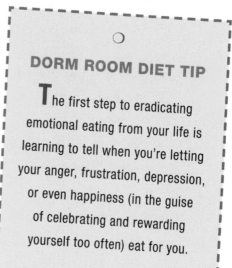

DORM ROOM DIET TIP

The first step to eradicating emotional eating from your life is learning to tell when you're letting your anger, frustration, depression, or even happiness (in the guise of celebrating and rewarding yourself too often) eat for you.

The key to meeting these challenges, without relying on food, is to understand that most of them are emotional and psychological in nature, and center around being uncomfortable with yourself. What's important to acknowledge is that college also offers a zillion ways for you to feel joy and find support systems. So, join a club, find a hobby that you love, make new friends, get a job. I'm sure you'll find, as my friends and I did, that having these outlets often provides an opportunity for social connection that leaves you feeling happy, fulfilled, and supported. Having good friends around who want what's best for you is a crucial step toward solidifying a stable environment in which you can really begin the process of adopting a healthy lifestyle. But if you don't know how to distinguish between emotional eating and biological hunger, it's hard to prevent yourself from getting stuck in a wicked cycle of eating for the wrong reasons.

The first step to eradicating emotional eating from your life is learning to tell when you're letting your anger, frustration, depression, or even happiness (in the guise of celebrating and rewarding yourself too often) eat for you. Here's how to recognize if you're hungry for something other than food:

➤ **You feel like food has control over you; you can't stop yourself from eating.**

➤ **You can't stop thinking about food, even right after you've eaten.**

➤ **Whenever you experience a lot of stress, hurt, or depression, or when something really great happens, your first reaction is to let food ease the pain or celebrate the joy.**

If these descriptions sound like they fit your relationship with food, it's up to you to stop the self-sabotage. By accepting the fact that emotional eating can never really solve any of your problems—more often it creates new ones—the temptation to "feed" your emotions might be lessened the next time you are in a difficult place. This was the case for Audrey, now twenty-six, who battled bulimia for six years before finally being able to quit the purging habit that nearly killed her.

Audrey, 26

I WAS ALWAYS an overweight child. From the time I can remember, I would go to the supermarket and my mom would let me have any candy or cookie I wanted, and I wanted them all. Both my mother and father were large individuals, so I thought I was supposed to be big, too. The kids in my elementary school quickly let me know that I was an "elephant-girl," not normal and not pretty and not liked. I was so ashamed of the way I looked, and I couldn't escape the teasing until I got home from school, where my parents would be waiting to comfort me with love and lots of sweets.

By the time I got to high school I had grown to 165 pounds on my slight 5' 4" build. Once, a girl in my class named Olivia asked me if I would like to go shopping with her. I lunged at the opportunity to spend time with a normal girl my age. After we shopped for her, she somehow convinced me to try on a pair of pants that I knew wouldn't fit. Ever since I was twelve, I had been shopping in women's stores, even in maternity stores sometimes. But I was too embarrassed to tell her that, so I pulled and tugged and tried to squeeze myself into pants that would never fit. She was more embarrassed than I was and apologized profusely for making me try them on, but the damage was done. When I got home that night, I went straight to the pantry, wolfed down an entire package of cookies, and got into bed, feeling sick and mortified. For fifteen minutes I sobbed into my pillow and thought about how fat, and hideous, and miserable I was and how there was nothing I could do about it. Then it dawned on me: I could keep eating as much as I wanted, as long as I got rid of the food afterward. I decided to do something about my life. I went to the bathroom, took out my toothbrush and made myself physically sick.

My mother heard me heaving in the bathroom and came rushing in to see what I was doing. She was appalled at the vision of me kneeling in front of the toilet, toothbrush in hand, eyes watery, and knuckles cut (from my teeth). She pulled me up and took me into my bedroom and we had a long discussion about how I was "beautiful inside and out" and "didn't need to fit in by making myself sick." I did a good job of convincing my mother that I had seen the error of my ways, but all that had changed was how I planned to hide my bulimia. (Yes, from the first day I wanted to be a bulimic, because I wanted desperately to fit in with a group somewhere.)

From freshman until senior year of high school, I would eat and purge, eat and purge. At school, I could just sneak into a private bathroom in the far corner of the school that nobody used. At home, I kept a bucket in my closet that I would empty directly into the Dumpster in back of our house. At first, I was worried my mother would see the cuts on my knuckles, but as I got "better" at purging, I learned how to use only my stomach muscles to send myself into convulsions.

I lost weight quickly at first and then, as my body started to adjust to the absence of food, and the nutrients it carries, my basal metabolism slowed and I lost weight more slowly. My teeth began to get yellow. I had sallow skin and acne sometimes and my breath was always rank, but I could see that people weren't staring at me in the hallways anymore, or making elephant noises when I walked past. The positive response of people not noticing me, rather than making fun, boosted my confidence that I had made the right choice.

But then I got to college. It became very difficult to find secret, private places where I could purge my food. I shared a tiny room with a workaholic roommate who was always in the dorm and we shared a bathroom with eight other girls. I would sneak off to other buildings, even once resorting to using a men's toilet, but this got too difficult to keep up, especially since my roommate began to suspect something. She would drop subtle hints about "something smelling like vomit," but I didn't care that she knew. I had to keep up the purging; otherwise, I would become the elephant again.

I was feeling more confident and secure in myself: my roommate and I were friends, even if she did think that I had a problem, and we decided to live together for a second year. I joined the stand-up comedy club at my university, and started to date a boy. I finally felt like I had things under control in my life. Until one day my legs locked while I was crossing the street and I fell over, almost being hit by an oncoming car. I was taken to the emergency room to be checked out. The doctors were searching around for a reason why a presumably healthy young woman would just collapse in the middle of the street. They stumbled upon my potassium reading, which was 1.9. The expected level for an average, functioning adult is 3.5. A level around 2.5 can be treated with pills; anything lower than 2.3 has to be treated with an IV. I had deprived my body of so many nutrients that it was actually shutting down, a symptom of which was muscle cramping. My body tried to reject the IV fluids and I swelled up overnight: I went from a size 6 to a size 10 in twelve hours. The doctors recognized my low potassium levels and adverse reaction to the IV fluids (since they flooded my body with nutrients I had been depriving it of for so long) as symptoms of an eating disorder and recommended that I see a therapist.

My boyfriend, who had come with me to the emergency room, didn't know what was going on but had overheard something about an eating disorder. I had to tell him about my problem. I couldn't stand the possibility of losing this person who I was growing to love so much. He told me that I could not expect him to love me if I didn't love myself. He had never said he loved me before, and hearing him talk about wanting to love me but not being able to because I didn't love myself was a true wake-up call. I realized I had to give up my crutch, my dependence on bulimia, if I wanted to regain myself.

I scheduled an appointment with a local therapist. It felt really good to have someone listen to me and understand why I could have felt so completely helpless in high school and at home. We talked about how the skinny girl I saw in the mirror that day was not what I thought the real me looked like: the real me was fat and awkward and uncomfortable. We began working on confidence-building exercises that helped me to regain some sort of self-love. After my fourth session, I got up the courage to call my parents and tell them about my problem and what had happened. With my family, my boyfriend, and my roommate aware of my problem, I had a constant support system to guard against the impulses to go back to purging. I kept seeing the therapist weekly for another two months, until I felt strong enough to join a support group instead.

I knew that I did not want to go back to being obese, nor could I go back to bulimia, so I started eating small, healthy portions. I even made it to the gym twice a week. At first, my body reacted horribly to my new routine: it swelled up from water retention and my clothing size fluctuated daily. It took months for my digestive system to be able to process food properly again. But I could not bear the thought of letting everyone I loved, and who truly loved me in return, down again. With the support of my family and friends, I was able to escape the clutches of my eating disorder. It is by no means a completed process, but I feel confident that with continued support (my boyfriend and I are now engaged, so he will keep on being my number one support system) I can succeed.

Audrey's story shows how needing to be loved and accepted drove her to adopt perilous habits. It took a near fatal event to get her there, but she was finally able to share her secret and become open to love, both from other people and from herself. Once she was able to do this, she could begin to address her emotional eating problems. Now she is in a place of recovery, with great prospects for success. While I certainly hope you never have to experience the severe emotional and physical pain Audrey endured, if you do, or anyone you know does, it is crucial that you seek professional assistance.

ANTIDOTES FOR EMOTIONAL EATING

- Whenever you feel like eating instead of dealing with the source of your emotions, take five deep breaths to clear your head and then take ten minutes to write out all your feelings, why you feel the way you do, and what your ideal solution would be.

- Talk to friends. Having people to listen to her problems and help her work through them got Audrey on the path to recovery. Sometimes, all you need is some sympathy and reassurance to help you deal with any stress or problem life presents.

- Separate emotional hunger or longing from the physical variety by getting involved in an activity that will provide outside support: it can be a tension-release activity, such as an exercise or yoga class, or a social activity, like a knitting or book club.

- If you still want to eat after you've taken the time to confront your emotions, you may be genuinely hungry. Have a glass of water and wait a few minutes and if the hunger persists, have something healthful to eat, like a handful of almonds, an apple, or some yogurt.

TAKING STOCK

So much of our emotional eating comes from being dissatisfied with our appearance. Try to be accepting of the beautiful body you've been given and learn to take care of it. It takes patience and commitment to become the healthiest, sexiest person you're capable of being, so try not to rush the process. Get informed about where you are now in terms of your body's needs, and decide on some realistic goals for the next several months, or even years. As a first step, answer the questions in the little inventory below.

1. **HOW TALL ARE YOU?**

2. **HOW MUCH DO YOU WEIGH?**

3. **WHERE DO YOU FIT ON THE CHART ON PAGE 49?** These widely used weight ranges are based on Metropolitan Life Insurance Company tables that were developed from figures on low mortality rates, not necessarily optimum health. Therefore, you should aim for the lower to middle region within these ranges, as this is a more accurate reflection of a healthy weight for your height and build. Another easy way to determine the lower end of the range is that a five-foot-tall woman should weigh 100 pounds; add 5 pounds for each additional inch over five feet.

Weight Chart for Women

Height	Small Frame	Medium Frame	Large Frame
4'10"	100–110	108–120	117–131
4'11"	101–112	110–123	119–134
5'0"	103–115	112–126	122–137
5'1"	105–118	115–129	125–140
5'2"	108–121	118–132	128–144
5'3"	111–124	121–135	131–148
5'4"	114–127	124–138	134–152
5'5"	117–130	127–141	137–156
5'6"	120–133	130–144	140–160
5'7"	123–136	133–147	143–164
5'8"	126–139	136–150	146–167
5'9"	129–142	139–153	149–170
5'10"	132–145	142–156	152–173
5'11"	135–148	145–159	155–176
6'0"	138–151	148–162	158–179

4. DO YOU EAT BREAKFAST?

5. HOW MANY MEALS A DAY DO YOU EAT OUT OF A BOX (i.e., not freshly prepared)?

6. HOW MANY APPLE-SIZED SERVINGS OF FRUIT DO YOU EAT DAILY?

7. HOW MANY HANDFUL-SIZED SERVINGS OF VEGGIES DO YOU EAT DAILY?

8. HOW MANY PALM-SIZED SERVINGS OF PROTEIN (MEAT, EGGS, NUTS) DO YOU EAT DAILY?

9. HOW MANY OUNCES OF WATER DO YOU DRINK DAILY?

10. HOW MANY HOURS DO YOU WORK OUT PER WEEK?

Compare your answers to questions 4 through 10 with the following "ideal" answers.

4. YES, I EAT A BREAKFAST, EVEN IF IT'S ONLY A PIECE OF FRUIT ON THE WAY OUT THE DOOR.

5. 1 OR NONE

6. 3

7. 5

8. 2–3

9. HALF OF YOUR BODY WEIGHT (IN POUNDS) IN OUNCES. FOR EXAMPLE, IF YOU WEIGH 150 POUNDS, YOU SHOULD BE DRINKING 75 OUNCES OF WATER DAILY.

10. 3–5 HOURS WEEKLY

Now, depending on your answer to question 3, you may have a lot or a little work to do. Because I do not advocate any sort of strict, pound-shedding diet in this book, you can expect to drop a pound or two a week until your body reaches a weight when it is in equilibrium and can burn the number of calories you consume daily without weight loss or gain. In order to find out if you're consuming the right number of calories to reach that equilibrium, we need to calculate your Basal Metabolic Rate (BMR).

WHAT'S YOUR NUMBER?

Your BMR is the number of calories your body burns daily without your having to do anything. Your body uses around 75 percent of the calories you eat each day just to maintain life and perform basic functions. You expend energy just to breathe, build new red and white blood cells, tone your muscles, pump blood throughout the body, think, raise or lower your body temperature—even while you're sleeping. Any activity you do in addition to these natural functions also requires fuel in the form of calories.

If you eat more calories than your body metabolism needs daily, you will gain weight. There are 3,500 calories in every pound of body fat. That means that if you eat 500 calories more per day than your body needs, you will gain one pound every week.

Your individual BMR depends on:

GENDER: Men generally have greater muscle mass and a lower body fat percentage. This means they have a higher basal metabolic rate, as muscle burns more calories per pound than fat does.

GENES: Some people are born with faster metabolisms, some with slower metabolisms; this genetic metabolic fact cannot be changed. However, building lean muscle does increase your BMR, so even if you don't have a naturally fast metabolism, you can rev it up it into the fast lane with proper exercise.

AGE: BMR declines with age. After age twenty, it drops about 2 percent per decade.

EXERCISE: Physical exercise influences body weight by burning calories, but it also helps raise your BMR by building extra lean muscle tissue, so you burn more calories all day and all night.

BODY FAT PERCENTAGE: The lower your percentage of body fat, the higher your BMR; the lower body fat percentage in the average male body is one reason why men generally have a 10 to 15 percent higher BMR than women. Unfair but true!

DIET: Starvation, eating disorders, or an abrupt calorie reduction can dramatically reduce BMR by up to 30 percent! Restrictive, low-calorie weight-loss diets may cause your BMR to drop by as much as 20 percent, because your body goes into starvation mode and will try to preserve itself by holding on to all the energy that comes into your body (which is stored as fat). Thus, if you don't eat breakfast or lunch but then eat dinner, just because you've taken in fewer calories than usual over the course of the day it doesn't mean you'll lose weight. If your body thinks it is starving (which is the normal response when it doesn't receive any food for a prolonged period of time), chances are it will try to hold on to any calories it does receive in the form of fat. You need to feed your body small meals and/or snacks at regular intervals throughout the day to make sure that your blood sugar is regulated and your body knows that more food is on the way. Eating as soon as you wake up is also a good idea because it kicks your metabolism into high gear (your metabolism drops while you sleep) and makes sure your BMR stays stable.

Most BMR calculators that you find on the Internet use something called the Harris-Benedict formula to calculate BMR based on total body weight, height, age, and gender. This particular method was developed around 1919, but it is still a good indicator of approximately how many calories you'll need daily. Because it does not take into account a *lean body mass* component, however, it tends to underestimate the caloric needs of extremely muscular people and overestimate the needs of extremely overweight (obese) people. But if you don't fall in either of these two extreme categories, you can calculate your approximate daily caloric needs using the steps below.

The Harris-Benedict Formula

MEN: BMR = 66 + (6.23 x weight in pounds) + (12.7 x height in inches) − (6.8 x age in years)

WOMEN: BMR = 655 + (4.35 x weight in pounds) + (4.7 x height in inches) − (4.7 x age in years)

Example:

You are female

You are 19 years old

You weigh 130 pounds

You are 5'6" tall

Your BMR = 655 + 565 + 310 − 89 = 1441 calories/day

Activity Multiplier

SEDENTARY = BMR x 1.2 (little or no exercise, sitting, driving, reading, sleeping)

LIGHT ACTIVITY = BMR x 1.375 (light exercise, walking, working out 1–3 days/week)

MODERATELY ACTIVE = BMR x 1.55 (moderate exercise/working out 1hr+, 3–5 days/week)

VERY ACTIVE = BMR x 1.725 (hard exercise/working out 1hr+, 6–7 days/week)

EXTREMELY ACTIVE = BMR x 1.9 (sports practice or a physical job, or working out 1hr+, twice daily)

Example:

Your BMR is 1441 calories per day

Your activity level is moderately active (work out 3–5 times per week)

Your activity factor is 1.55

Your Total Energy Needs = 1.55 x 1441 = 2233 calories/day

Your "total energy needs" means the number of calories you burn daily. To lose weight, you need to eat fewer calories than your body burns daily. To gain weight, eat more calories than your body burns daily.

Keeping the amount of calories you ingest daily below or close to your BMR number and getting your answers to the self-inventory section as close to the ideal answers as possible will help accelerate this process of reaching equilibrium. But how to go about getting all the portion sizes and servings right? That's the subject of Step 3.

STEP 3

GET STARTED

Healthy Eating 101

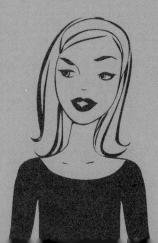

" I've struggled with my weight since I was little. When I got into high school, I decided to try a diet, like every other girl I knew, but I could never stick to it. I'd be 'good' for a few days, maybe even a week, only to go off track at a friend's birthday party or another get-together. I'd get so down on myself that it would take me another few days to convince myself that I was not a pathetic person with no willpower and get back on track—but the choices were so limiting that I'd soon be off track again. My self-esteem plummeted and my weight soared as a result of my inability to stick to these plans."

—DAKOTA, 18

HOW WOULD YOU like to be able to eat anything you want, wherever you like, and still be able to lose weight and look great? No calorie counting, no food scales, no strict guidelines that make it impossible for you to eat anything besides grapefruit. Just you in control of what you eat. Sounds amazing, right?

The eating system we'll talk about in this chapter is a plan for life, not a trendy quick fix that will more than likely backfire in time. Underlying this plan is the principle that *eating should be enjoyable*. Food is meant for fuel, but good eating habits go a long way toward giving you boundless energy, mental brilliance, and a youthful glow—not to mention that they help your body fend off osteoporosis, diabetes, cancer, and other debilitating diseases, all of which have been linked to poor nutrition. Now that's something to feel good about.

Recent studies have shown that the mere mention of the word "diet" triggers a stress response in a woman's body, causing increased levels of anxiety and insecurity. This could be because we typically use the word "diet" to refer to is an eating plan full of restrictions and extremes, in which pain and self-hatred are the rules, and failure is always just around the corner. These diets lure people in with promises of rapid weight loss with just "one simple step." That step generally includes cutting out carbs, cutting out fat, cutting out fruit or veggies, or only eating certain things at certain times, and there is never anything "simple" about it. These diets can assure you results *if you can stick to their strict guidelines*. The thing is, in the long run, these extreme regimens can actually make you *gain* weight. How's that? Allow me to explain.

FATKINS:
HOW NO CARBS MAKE YOU FAT

Your body requires nutrition from three macronutrient groups: carbohydrates, proteins, and fats. (Vitamins, minerals, essential fatty acids, and amino acids are micronutrients that your body can't make itself and that you need to take as supplements or get through food. We'll talk more about micronutrients in Step 7.) Carbohydrates are made from plants that contain sugar, starch, or fiber, such as refined sugar, grains, and even fruits and veggies (think: bagels, brown rice, and potatoes). Because they store energy, carbs act as the fuel for your body, providing it with energy it can use immediately. But if you don't use the energy you consume, your body stores this extra fuel as fat. So if you eat too many carbs and don't get enough physical exercise, you store lots of fat around your body.

Protein forms the building blocks for your body's muscles, and muscles burn fat. Lean muscle burns fat by controlling your BMR (the basal metabolic rate we discussed in Step 2), the number of calories you burn when you're doing nothing. Each pound of lean muscle burns 50 calories every day without your having to lift so much as a finger. If you start losing muscle, your basal metabolism will go down and your body will burn fewer calories per day, which could mean weight gain for you.

Whenever a diet suggests that you drastically limit or even halt your intake of one of the macronutrient groups, your body has to adjust the source and use of its energy and fuel.

For instance, low-carb diets, such as the famous Atkins plan, initially help you to lose weight because you are limiting the amount of *glucose* (a simple carb) entering your body. Whenever you eat carbs, your digestive system breaks up larger molecules, such as starch and fiber, into simpler sugars, or *glucose*; this sugar circulates in your bloodstream, and is called blood sugar. It is transported to all the different cells in your body, where it is either immediately used for cell functions or stored as *glycogen* in your muscles and liver. When all the glucose in your bloodstream is depleted, your body begins to break down glycogen, since it is easier to convert for fuel than fat or protein. But your body stores only so much glycogen (about enough for one strenuous workout). When this store is finished, it needs to be replenished by eating carbs—which can't happen if you aren't eating any. In addition, with every molecule of glycogen that is released from your muscles for energy, three molecules of water are also released. Loss of this "water weight" accounts for a lot of that initial weight

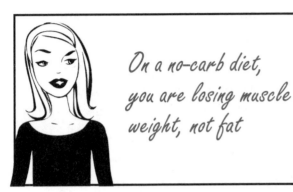

On a no-carb diet, you are losing muscle weight, not fat

loss you see at the beginning of low-carb diets. Losing glycogen stores and water will cause your muscles to shrink (lowering your basal metabolism) so that, while it may seem as if you are losing a tremendous amount of weight in the first weeks of a no-carb diet,

it's important to keep in mind that *you are losing muscle weight, not fat,* and that, long term, your ability to burn calories is declining.

Did I mention the depression and fatigue that comes with cutting out carbs? Because carbs are your brain's main fuel, cutting them out may cause you to feel slow and foggy, and the lack of immediate fuel reserves will make you tired and less likely to exercise. Also, a lack of carbs lowers the level of *serotonin*, the "happy" neurotransmitter in your brain, making many dieters depressed and grouchy. In fact, some studies have shown that low-carb plans can cause mood swings that can lead to emotional binge eating. How's that for a vicious cycle?

Good luck losing weight when you're leading a sedentary life (and your BMR is burning off fewer calories than before you started because of muscle loss) and you're increasingly depressed and longing for that carb fix you can't have. End result: failed weight loss and diminished health in the long run.

On some level, all fad diets are restrictive eating plans that have adverse effects on your body. You can't survive following these regimens for the rest of your life, or you'll go crazy. And, since most of these programs work because of calorie deprivation and water loss and not because of any inherent fat-zapping quality in the "magic" foods they allow, why not choose to follow a system that lets you make all the choices, eat a balanced amount from all the food groups, and not have to worry about rules and regulations?

If you're ready to be in the driver's seat of your eating, you first need to understand what different foods do to your body. There are five main categories of food from which you can choose for optimal mental and physical health. I've collaborated with several doctors and nutritionists to compile the brief summaries below from the vast amount of information available.

SIMPLE AND COMPLEX CARBOHYDRATES

Most breakfast foods that come already prepared (such as toaster strudel, doughnuts, etc.) are *simple carbohydrates*, made up almost entirely of refined, processed flour and sugar. The easiest way I know to remember what simple carbohydrates are is to think about the word "simple."

"Simple" is used to connote the ease with which your body can extract the sugars from the carbohydrates you have just eaten. The reason it is so easy for your body to get these sugars is because machines have already done most of the work for you. A whole grain is the unprocessed grain kernel. This means it has its hard, outer husk and seed still intact. This hard material is the stuff that is removed when grains are processed by machines—making it easier for your body to get at the sugars inside the grain. Any food that is made up primarily of grain (corn, wheat, or rice, for example), in which the seeds and husks have been removed by a machine, is already halfway digested for you. When you eat the regurgitated food of machines, you aren't getting all the nutrients and fiber grains naturally supply (a lot of which is stored in the husk and seed that the machines removed). Not only do you need these things to stay energized, healthy, and regular (fiber helps you to have a smooth move, if you catch my drift), but they also help you feel fuller on less food.

As soon as you swallow that first bite of a doughnut, you experience a sudden leap in your blood sugar level, giving you an instant boost of energy. But your body quickly compensates with an output of *insulin* (the hormone that metabolizes carbohydrates and regulates blood sugar), lowering your blood sugar level and storing the excess sugar as fat, which leaves you tired and craving more sugar to give you another energy boost. Sounds an awful lot like the effects of morphine or heroin on the body: a brief high followed by a debilitating slump that leaves the victim desperately foraging for her next hit (or bite, in this case). The vicious cycle continues because simple carbohydrates don't keep you full for long and leave you craving more of the same. So you are never full, always tired and lethargic, and aren't getting proper nutrients because all you can think about eating are processed, sugary, fake foods: simple carbs, in a nutshell.

On the other hand, minimally processed treats such as oatmeal, whole grain or whole wheat bread, and granola bars in which you can see the hunky grains and seeds are known as *complex carbohydrates.* Always go for brown over white, but understand that some brown breads are just a company's attempts to get you to think you are eating healthfully by coloring white bread brown; stick with items clearly labeled "whole grain" in which you can see the grains. It is much more difficult, much more *complex,* for your body to get the sugar out of these babies because it first has to break down the fiber (the grainy part you can see) surrounding the sugars. Because this process takes more energy and time, you stay full longer and don't get hungry as quickly as when you eat simple carbohydrates. And, since your body is extracting the sugars out of your oatmeal in small increments, your blood sugar does not experience sudden leaps and falls, so you don't have a short energy burst followed by a long slump, and you don't get cravings. Whole grains also supply the full benefit of the nutrients these foods have to offer. See the lists at the end of this chapter for other examples of simple and complex carbs that are easy to find on or near college campuses.

THE RIGHT FRUITS AND VEGGIES

Any fruit or vegetable is an excellent choice as a snack or part of a meal. These foods are a yummy source of the many vitamins and minerals that you need to survive, not to mention look your best (the amino acids and nutrients they contain improve your complexion and give you a radiant glow). Fruits and veggies are indeed carbohydrates, and although fruits do contain sugar, this sugar is ingested along with natural proteins and fibers. Fruits are considered complex carbs, and, as we discussed in the last section, complex carbs are a great and healthy source of energy. They're also a terrific source of fiber (to fill you up and keep you satisfied longer), as well as various vitamins and minerals.

There are so many options to choose from in this food category, you really can't go wrong. Of course it's best to stick to whole, fresh, unadulterated fruits and veggies since, for example, dried fruits are loaded with concentrated sugar and potato chips give up their status as a vegetable during the second frying. Baked, steamed, grilled, or lightly sautéed vegetables are fine, if you want something other than raw. A good rule of thumb is that any dark green, leafy vegetable (spinach, kale), crucifer (broccoli, cauliflower), or vine-growing vegetable (peas) is low in sugar and rich in vitamins and minerals. Any root vegetable (potatoes, carrots) has a bit more sugar in it. With fruits, your taste buds can be a very useful guide. Fruits that taste the sweetest probably have the most sugar in them. But even the sweetest fruits don't come close to the sugar content of a candy bar, so don't sweat it if you go a little wild one day with the grapes.

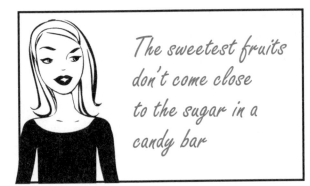

The sweetest fruits don't come close to the sugar in a candy bar

A word of caution: a glass of fruit juice, especially artificially flavored or concentrated versions, has nearly as much sugar as a can of soda. Watch for the words "sugar added" (usually in small type) on the bottle. And beware of the terms "juice drink" and "cocktail." Generally these beverages contain low amounts of real fruit juice—as low as 5 percent. For the most part, try to stick to water and 100 percent natural juices. (One of my favorite sweet fixes is a glass of sparkling water spiked with real fruit juice and a wedge of lime, if you have it.)

While some dietitians recommend diet sodas to satisfy a sweet tooth, some artificial sweeteners in diet drinks, such as aspartame and saccharin, have been linked with allergies and even cancers; in addition, the carbonation leaches calcium out of your bones. This is particularly worrisome for young women, since we have a greater likelihood of developing osteoporosis than men do. Unfortunately, the sparkling water and club soda I'm so fond of have the same carbonation, so I really try to moderate my sparkling drink intake.

Even worse, new studies are showing that your body may process artificial sugar the same way it does regular sugar. Part of the science behind this suggests that because your body is a smart, well-tuned machine, when it tastes something sweet, it expects to receive some actual sugar. In diet sodas, there is no real sugar, and your body is confused because it was anticipating a leap in blood sugar that never happened. As a result, it overcompensates and tells you that you need to eat something that can provide this real sugar (you may know this as the craving for chocolate or some other simple carb after you enjoy a soda—which might explain why popcorn and candy are available at movie theaters to accompany your "refreshing beverage"). Moreover, researchers at Purdue University have found that consumption of artificial sweeteners caused rats to overeat, perhaps because the body's natural way of regulating hunger is thrown out of balance as a result of the chemicals used to make artificially sweetened foods and drinks taste like something they are not. The point is, don't think you're doing yourself any favors when you skip calories and opt for diet sodas: you may actually increase your likelihood of weight gain by altering your brain chemistry and metabolism.

In general, whenever you need a snack and it isn't really time for a meal, fruits and veggies are the right foods to choose. Grab a nectarine or a pear, or some carrots, celery, or peppers to tide you over until dinner. I love to have radishes with a little salt or some yogurt with fresh dill if I have it (you can also go for a low-sugar, low-fat dressing), or, if I'm feeling a little fruitier, I'll have apple slices with peanut butter. All these things are easy to find on or around campus and, assuming you keep the dip and peanut butter to a reasonable amount, these snacks shouldn't total more than 200 calories.

OVEREATING WITH SODA

While we're on the topic of soda and weight gain, I thought I'd take the opportunity to explain a bit about how your body regulates appetite. Basically, hunger and satiety are controlled by a complex mix of hormones. What some science is now uncovering is that pure calories alone may play only a partial role in creating the feeling of being full. This is especially important when we look at how your body responds to solid food versus caloried beverages (anything other than water, basically).

One of the most important hormones you should know about is called ghrelin, and it is responsible for signaling your body that it is time to eat. When you eat simple carbs (remember, these are food and drinks where it is very easy for your body to access the calories and sugar because there is limited fiber, protein, or fat), they cause a huge blood sugar spike. Your body then releases insulin to break down the sugar it perceives in the body, but overcompensates because the spike was so immediate and sudden, eliminating all the sugar and then some so that you have low blood sugar. Your body now recognizes the need to replenish sugar supplies and tells you to eat something by releasing ghrelin and other hormones, which is why you're hungry again so soon after eating a meal of purely simple carbohydrates (the not-so-happy meal).

The level of ghrelin output in your body soars before you eat something, and drops after you've eaten, but we're now learning that what you ate to satiate your hunger plays a big role in how long it takes for ghrelin levels to rise again. For instance, when you eat a piece of whole grain toast with peanut butter, the level of ghrelins drops for several hours, but this is not true even if you slurp down a 24-ounce soda with twice the calories. Even if the bubbles help to fill you up temporarily, you'll most likely be hungry again soon. Things like chewing sensation, smell, and taste affect how hungry we feel, but our expectations also play a role. For instance, people perceive soup as a meal, even though it is liquid, so the disparity in ghrelin levels after you eat soup versus solid food is minimal. The science of how what you eat affects how hungry you are is constantly evolving, but it provides added incentive to make sure you are limiting the number of empty calories coming in from simple carbohydrates, and especially beverages.

LIKE BUTTA!
THE DAIRY YOUR BODY NEEDS

Lean dairy foods, such as low-fat or fat-free varieties, offer a slew of benefits to the body. Everyone has seen the milk mustache ads advocating the wonders of this simple, accessible drink. Along with other dairy products such as yogurt, cheese, even ice cream (albeit, the sugar probably isn't worth the nutritional benefits), milk is a good source of vitamin D, calcium, and other bone-strengthening nutrients. (You can also get vitamin D from sun exposure, though milk offers it without the threat of skin cancer.)

Recent studies have shown that people who consume calcium-rich foods, such as milk and other dairy products, lose weight more quickly (especially in the midsection around your belly) and are better able to keep that weight off than people on the same diet who aren't getting enough calcium. It's important to keep in mind, however, that the people who lose weight by consuming dairy are probably not drinking whole milk or eating full-fat yogurt. Simply switching from whole milk (which is about 3.25 percent fat) to 2 percent milk (which is 1.5 to 1.8 percent fat) or skim (0.1 percent fat) significantly limits the amount of fat you are ingesting—without limiting all the other good stuff you get from milk. The same applies for most yogurts, ice creams, and other dairy foods. I usually opt for some fat because I find it helps me stay fuller for longer and is worth the relatively small indulgence.

There is, however, one area in which low fat isn't necessarily better for your health: butter. When people want to eat butter but are trying to limit their fat intake, they often switch to margarine. This is not a good choice because margarine contains *hydrogenated* fats, the kind that will stick to

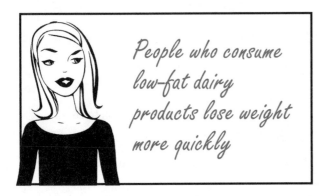

People who consume low-fat dairy products lose weight more quickly

the lining of your various tubes, especially those in and around your heart, which can lead to artery clogs and heart attacks later in life. The best plan with butter is just to go for the real stuff and eat it sparingly; don't switch over to a completely artificial substitute that may hurt you more than the few extra fat calories in butter.

Weight loss aside, you need calcium and vitamin D to ensure proper growth, strong bones, and a robust immune system. Getting this calcium is especially important since, according to *Time* magazine, the average teen gets 10 to 15 percent of her daily calories from soda and, as I mentioned earlier, carbonation leaches calcium out of bones. In this way, we are putting ourselves at unnecessary risk for osteoporosis, or bone thinning. (Trust me, this is one place you don't want to be thin.) That can of soda doesn't seem so refreshing now, does it?

MUSCLE FOOD
IN MODERATION: PROTEIN

If there's one macronutrient group we don't have to worry about getting enough of, it's protein. Americans consume more protein than the people of any other nation (about *five times* as much protein as we need), but often it's the wrong type of protein, that is, protein that is accompanied by tons of fat. Hamburgers, chicken nuggets, ham and cheese: we love our meats, but we also love to smother them in creamy sauces, fry them in butter or oil, or combine them with animal fats to improve the taste.

Of course, there are good things that come from eating protein. Proteins provide the building blocks, called amino acids and polypeptides (don't worry, there's no quiz on this), of all muscle tissue. Eating enough protein keeps your muscles strong and powerful and your basal metabolism high. Protein is also your "brain food." Because your brain is one big muscle, not getting enough protein can hurt brain function. For example, the different parts of your brain communicate to one another through neurotransmitters, chemical signals that require polypeptides to form. A deficiency in protein can mean that brain functioning suffers.

On the other hand, eating too much protein, as we do in the United States, can also do us harm. The body uses protein to make DNA, RNA, and muscle, the basic building blocks of all body functions. Any protein the body doesn't use for these processes is flushed out as waste. During this process, protein is broken down in the liver to ammonia, a highly toxic chemical. Your liver then turns the ammonia into urea, a precursor to urine, which has to be excreted by the kidneys. When more than 15 percent of your daily calories come from protein, the strain on your liver and kidneys can become too much to bear. Under this strain, your liver and kidneys enlarge and the kidneys change their physiology. This may cause, among other ailments, significant calcium loss, pulled from your bones into your urine. If this sounds to you like another good reason to avoid super high-protein, low-carb diets, you're right.

The average person should only be having about three small (palm-sized, half-inch-thick) portions of protein per day. But *where* you get your protein is also important to take into consideration. Meat proteins often have high levels of sulfur-containing amino acids, which contribute to calcium loss, whereas vegetable proteins do not. So, eating kidney beans (26 percent protein) would be preferable to beef (also 26 percent protein) if you don't want to start losing calcium in your urine. Chicken breast and beef have about the same level of protein, but skinless chicken breast has about 3 grams of fat, while even 95 percent lean ground beef has more than 5 grams per serving. Good sources of protein are lean meats, fish, poultry, and eggs, in addition to legumes (lentils, peas, beans, and peanuts) and some other vegetables. Vegetarians, like me, can get plenty of protein from beans, legumes, tofu, and, of course, vegetables. In any case, you should try to get some protein in at every meal, especially because it staves off hunger and can keep you from overeating—but keep in mind that you should not be eating meat more than once a day, so opt for those vegetable or egg sources. Some easy protein snacks include: a small handful of peanuts (18 percent protein), some carrots (10 percent protein), a slice of low-fat cheddar cheese (25 percent protein), or a slice of whole grain bread (16 percent protein) with peanut butter (18 percent protein).

THE SKINNY ON GOOD FATS (YES, THERE ARE GOOD ONES)

Shocking as it may sound, some fats are not only good for you, but are absolutely essential to proper brain function, good joint movement, lustrous hair, glowing skin, and shiny nails—not to mention pleasure in life and eating, since fats make things taste good. Fats fall into two categories: saturated and unsaturated. Saturated fats are solid at room temperature and can usually be found in animal tissues, while unsaturated fats are liquid at room temperature and are found in plants (we see them mostly in vegetable oils, such as canola and olive oil).

Your body can also synthesize its own fats from the carbohydrates you eat, as it needs to. The only fats it cannot make are certain unsaturated ones, which you have to get from food. These are called *essential fatty acids*

(EFA) or *omega fats*. EFAs are sometimes classified as omega-3s or omega-6s. (EFAs must be provided in the diet—the body cannot make them.) Omega-3s are the best for maintaining lean muscles, and waistlines, and can be found in flax products (including flaxseed oil or crushed flaxseeds) and in fatty cold-water fish, such as salmon, Chilean sea bass, and cod. Omega-3s should be consumed in equal proportion to omega-6s, but our society consumes about ten times more omega-6s, found in vegetable oils such as soybean and sunflower, which can result in water retention and weight gain. Try to get your consumption of omega-3 and omega-6 fats into balance by lowering your intake of vegetable oils (used in most processed, boxed goodies) and working olive oil and/ or flaxseed or cod liver oil (good sources of omega-3s) into your diet. I like to make sure I'm getting a good dose of omega-3 fats daily by taking two tablespoons of cod liver oil shaken into a shot of orange juice with breakfast (you can also take cod liver oil in pill form). Cod liver oil is available at any health store and can be stored in a mini fridge; the lemon-flavored varieties are more pleasant to take. I find this small step helps keep me feeling full until lunch and improves my brain function all day long (not to mention, leaves my skin, hair, and nails lustrous.

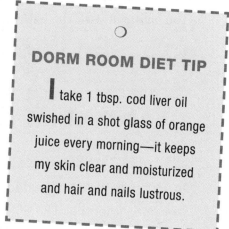

DORM ROOM DIET TIP

I take 1 tbsp. cod liver oil swished in a shot glass of orange juice every morning—it keeps my skin clear and moisturized and hair and nails lustrous.

Not only is eating a reasonable amount of good fats not bad for you, it can actually help you lose weight by maintaining healthy, lean muscle (keeping that basal metabolism we talked about high), and suppressing your appetite. Omega fats specifically work in two other ways to help you lose weight. First, they help your body unlock stored body fat so it can be burned for energy. (This is done through a process that involves balancing your body's ratio of *insulin,* the chemical signal that tells your body to store fat, and *glucagon,* the chemical signal that tells your body to burn fat.) And second, omega fats boost your body's metabolism, increasing the number of calories you burn daily. Keep in mind that overdoing any kind of fat, good or bad, is a silly move if you are trying to lose weight. But don't throw the baby out with the bathwater—the good fats need to stay in your diet.

FILL UP— AND SLIM DOWN—WITH FIBER

While fiber is not its own food group, it is an important component of many foods that you need to consume to make sure your digestive system functions smoothly. The fiber in foods helps you to stay full longer because it swells when it comes into contact with water. As this hydrated fiber passes through your intestines and bowel, it gently cleans the inside of the tract, making sure that you don't get any nasty growths or clots of garbage rotting in the crevices and bends of these organs.

Young women should be getting about 25 grams of fiber daily. You can easily get this amount in your diet by eating five servings of raw fruits and veggies and a bowl of high-fiber cereal (such as shredded wheat or raisin bran) daily. Complex carbs, such as brown rice and whole grain bread, are also good sources of fiber. You can also swallow the new and highly convenient pill forms of Metamucil (psyllium husks), a dietary fiber supplement taken fifteen minutes before lunch and dinner to help you feel full faster and make sure that any food you don't digest is easily passed from your body. Regardless of where you get your fiber (though you should try to make sure as much as possible comes from natural, whole foods), high fiber intake helps you lose weight by helping you feel full faster (so you don't overeat) and stay full longer (so you don't overeat again). Plus, it makes sure that you eliminate all the refuse quickly and easily, so you're not walking around bloated and uncomfortable.

SIZE DOES MATTER: PORTIONS

So how much of each of these different food categories should you be eating daily? Ideally, you will keep the amount of simple carbohydrates *very* low, or risk making the scale read very high. The number of servings of complex carbohydrates is not set in stone. A small serving (one that would fit in the palm of your hand) at every meal is plenty, but if you need more, simply increase you physical activity to balance the increased food consumption (you can't gain weight if you're burning the calories you eat). You should be having five to eight tennis-ball–size servings of fruits and/or veggies daily. With dairy, you want to keep to about two portions daily. Normally you can just go by the portion size indicated on the package of the dairy product, but be sure you read how many servings the package contains. In general, an ounce of cheese is about the size of a golf ball.

Red meat should be kept to a bare minimum, since even lean cuts are fatty. You should only consume a maximum of two fist-size servings per week. But you can have two servings of nonmeat lean protein per day (cheese, legumes, etc.) and one serving of meat protein. Also, a fistful of nuts a few times weekly, cod liver oil in the morning, and some olive oil thrown on your salad, is plenty of added fats. Don't forget that you are also getting fat from your low-fat dairy products, eggs, butter, cooking oils, and in other hidden components of the meal. Use the box on page 74 for an at-a-glance checklist.

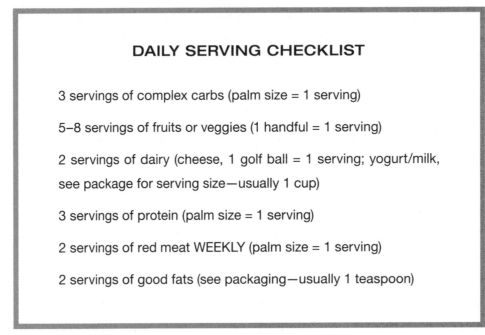

DAILY SERVING CHECKLIST

3 servings of complex carbs (palm size = 1 serving)

5–8 servings of fruits or veggies (1 handful = 1 serving)

2 servings of dairy (cheese, 1 golf ball = 1 serving; yogurt/milk, see package for serving size—usually 1 cup)

3 servings of protein (palm size = 1 serving)

2 servings of red meat WEEKLY (palm size = 1 serving)

2 servings of good fats (see packaging—usually 1 teaspoon)

WHAT, NO CALORIE COUNTING?

In this book, I don't talk about how many calories you should be consuming daily (except to use the BMR to give yourself a general window) because that number varies greatly from person to person, depending on how fast your individual metabolism works and how much exercise you get daily. The serving recommendations above are adequate for a 5'5" woman weighing 125 pounds. If you find that this is too much or too little food for your body type, adjust accordingly. Just follow this basic principle: if you need extra calories, they should come from complex carbohydrates and proteins, rather than fats. If you need fewer calories, eliminate one serving from the complex carbohydrate group and/or from fat or dairy. Also, be sure to keep in mind that, if you are an athlete or are expending large amounts of energy daily through vigorous exercise, you will need to increase the amount of energy (calories) you take in. As always, if you think you are not getting enough calories through your daily eating, you should consult a diet specialist who might suggest meal-supplementing drinks or nutritious snacks to boost your daily energy intake.

GRAB-AND-GO FOODS

Who says convenience foods have to be garbage? Below you will find a list of grab-and-go foods that you can either prepare quickly or just grab out of the box, which won't leave you in a sugar slump an hour later. These are some of the foods I was able to find easily at my college, either at the campus food store or at a nearby convenience store. Buying them regularly didn't break the bank. The ones that needed preparation involved merely adding hot water or using the small communal kitchen downstairs, and the perishable items were easy to store.

Complex Carbs

Cooked Cereals (look for at least 3 grams of fiber per serving)

These should be eaten plain or with sparing amounts of butter, milk, and/or sugar.

Instant or regular oatmeal, unflavored, unsweetened

Farina cereal, cooked

Oat bran, cooked

Cold Cereals

All cereals should be eaten dry or with 1 percent or skim milk. Try to avoid sweetened cereals or putting sugar on cereal.

Whole grain granola bars, with less than 150 calories and minimal added sugar

Whole grain cereals

All-Bran

All-Bran with extra fiber

All-Bran Buds

Chex, Multi-Bran or Wheat (and gluten-free varieties)

Fortified oat flakes

40% Bran Flakes

Flax & Fiber

Fruitful Bran

Granola, low fat, low sugar

Grape-Nuts

Mueslix

100% Bran

Raisin Bran (because raisins can be sugarcoated, a healthier choice would be to just add your own raisins to plain bran flakes)

Shredded Wheat, unfrosted

Special K

Total

Baked Goods

Multigrain bagel, plain or with low-fat/low-sugar toppings

Oat-bran bagel, plain or with low-fat/low-sugar toppings

Crackers, whole wheat, low fat

Melba toast

Breads:

Cracked wheat

High-fiber

Multigrain

Whole grain, any kind

Rye, light, or dark

The Best Fruits

Apples	Mangoes
Applesauce, unsweetened	Melon
Apricots	Nectarines
Bananas*	Oranges
Blackberries	Papaya*
Blueberries	Peaches*
Cherries	Pears
Cranberries	Pineapple
Figs	Plums
Grapefruit	Raspberries
Grapes	Strawberries
Kiwi	Tangelo
Lemon	Tangerines
Lime	Watermelon*

* *These fruits have more fruit sugar (fructose) than the rest and should be eaten in moderation. Remember, you should eat all fruit raw, whenever possible. Dried fruit has an abundance of condensed sugar, and stewed or packaged fruits often have had sugar added. If you can't store or don't like raw fruit, go for the dehydrated kind (for example, JustFruit bars) or have a little dried fruit with no sugar added.*

STOP-DROP-OR-ROLL

I have a category of food I call stop-drop-or-roll because they will make you tired, hungry, and fat if you eat too much of them. When you find yourself about to indulge, stop yourself, drop it, or prepare to roll. This list includes the culprits I found to be most tempting and readily available at my school, but you may find that your campus has its own unique temptations that you will have to deem unhealthy on your own.

Alcoholic beverages (beer, wine, liquor)

Cheese, full-fat

Fruit juice, concentrated or cocktail

Fried food of any kind

Meat, high-fat cuts (red meat should be eaten sparingly,
   no more than two 4-ounce [fist-size] servings per week)

Simple carbohydrates:

Bagel chips	Pies
Biscuits	Pretzels, not whole grain or whole wheat
Bread sticks	
Brownies	Toaster pastries
Cakes	Waffles
Cookies	White bread
Doughnuts	White rice
Pancakes	Sweet soft drinks

SOME CONTROVERSIAL ITEMS

Finally, I want to mention some controversial items that you're bound to encounter at school—you'll probably find students subsisting on them. Specifically, I'm going to go out on a limb and advocate drinking coffee, eating chocolate, and having bread (with olive oil) before a meal. Don't worry, it's not as crazy as it sounds!

Coffee

Despite school administrators' dire warnings that caffeine renders students incapable of concentrating or retaining information, somehow college students don't seem to give a hoot. Coffee and other caffeinated beverages seem to be the drink of choice for almost everyone (at least before the parties get under way). And guess what? A few doctors are actually on our side. Drs. Michael Roizen and Mehmet Oz (yes, my dad) in their book *You: The Owner's Manual* stress that drinking four six-ounce cups of caffeinated coffee daily is not harmful in the least, and, if anything, may slow the aging of your immune system; this means that your body stays youthful longer and is better able to function and protect itself against disease and sickness.

Now, this statement does not completely refute all the years of study on how caffeine can limit memorization abilities and concentration. Caffeine is a drug and can be physically addictive. Coffee stains your teeth and leaves you with rank breath (think crotchety history teacher), and caffeine can make you jumpy and can interfere with sleep. But, as long as you're not drinking more than four small cups a day and you aren't experiencing negative side effects, the most recent studies say you're good to go. Of course, when these doctors talk about drinking coffee, they mean black or with a little skim milk or 2 percent milk added—not sugar-loaded coffee smoothies or other fancy beverages with tons of sugar and full-fat milk or cream.

If coffee isn't your thing or you're trying to ease up on how much you drink, there are some alternatives that give you the same energy boost as the caffeine in coffee. Green and white teas have lesser concentrations of caffeine than coffee, so they might be better for those of you who need a little pick-me-up but don't want to be staring at your dorm room ceiling at 4 a.m. Green tea has the added benefit of being an antioxidant, so it keeps your immune system healthy and you looking and feeling younger, and it's also a natural appetite suppressant—it's practically a miracle drink.

You can also do a little exercise to wake up. If you feel safe, taking a brisk walk outside is a great way to exercise and get reenergized. Or, if leaving the premises isn't advisable, running up stairs and doing stretching and breathing exercises right in your dorm room can get the blood moving in your body and rush a fresh supply to the brain so you can continue cramming. Also, chocolate contains a caffeine-like compound, though not in very high amounts. If you really want a little chocolate and are looking for an excuse, it *can* help perk you up. And vitamin B_6, which you can take as a supplement (more on this in Step 7), will give you an energy boost just as an espresso would. So, you don't have to drink up to stay up!

Chocolate

A lot depends on the kind of chocolate you're eyeing. While "chocolate" imposters, like many milk chocolates, are made from flavored trans fats (mutilated fats that are terrible for your body) and have very little real cocoa content, real chocolate, the kind made from cocoa butter, is rich in flavonoids, special antioxidants that slow the aging process and reinforce your immune system. No doubt about it, chocolate is fattening, so it should be savored in moderation. But if you need a little pick-me-up—either to snap out of a yawning spree or an emotional slump, or to stave off those time-of-the-month cravings, a little piece of dark chocolate with at least 75 percent cocoa delivers. The more than four hundred chemicals in chocolate may positively affect your body's "happy" mood chemicals, including serotonin, endorphins, and even phenylethylamine, the body's chemical response to romance. Ooh-la-la!

Bread Before Meals

You may have thought you were doing yourself a service by asking the waiter to take away the basket of steaming, fresh-from-the-oven bread before it even touched the table. But studies prove that if you indulge in a small piece of whole wheat or whole grain bread dipped in some good fat (such as olive oil), rather than slathered with butter, before the meal you are less likely to overeat and will consume fewer total calories than if you had not eaten the bread. This is because it takes some time for your body to realize that you are eating and it is becoming full, so the more spaced out you can make your meal (e.g., having a piece of bread twenty minutes before your meal arrives, or even eating a piece of fruit on your way to the restaurant), the more likely your body is to recognize that it is becoming full and keep you from overeating. So, stop denying yourself that unsinful pleasure and have a piece.

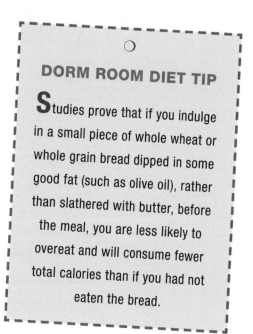

DORM ROOM DIET TIP

Studies prove that if you indulge in a small piece of whole wheat or whole grain bread dipped in some good fat (such as olive oil), rather than slathered with butter, before the meal, you are less likely to overeat and will consume fewer total calories than if you had not eaten the bread.

FIVE PRINCIPLES
FOR HEALTHY EATING

By now I hope you feel you know a lot more about *what* to eat at college. But even people who know everything about what to eat can fail to reach their goals if they eat too much, eat at the wrong times, or eat for the wrong reasons.

During our freshman year at college, my friends and I devised a list of five secrets or principles for controlling our weight. These little tricks, which become instinctual after you practice them for a while, made us much more aware of what and when we ate—and healthier because of it.

1. **ALWAYS HAVE BREAKFAST.** This ensures that your body won't go into starvation-preservation mode and also provides your body and brain with energy so you can be on top of your game. Don't forget it also revs up your metabolism for all-day calorie-burning power!

2. **DRINK HALF YOUR BODY WEIGHT IN OUNCES OF WATER DAILY, INCLUDING ONE GLASS BEFORE EVERY MEAL.** So, if you weigh 140 pounds, try to drink 70 ounces of water each day. It seems like a lot, but drinking a sufficient amount of water keeps your complexion clear and skin glowing, flushes toxins out of your body, aids in good digestion and healthy teeth, and suppresses appetite. Also, drinking a full glass of water right before bed helps prevent bags under your eyes, as this swelling is caused by an abundance of salt in the body; water flushes it out of your system.

3. **EAT AT LEAST EVERY THREE HOURS (THREE MEALS AND TWO SNACKS OF FRUIT OR VEGGIES).** This makes sure that you are fueled throughout the day so your body doesn't go into starvation-preservation mode. It also ensures that you won't be ravenous at any point in the day, making it less likely that you'll binge when you do eat or resort to eating something unhealthy just to put something in your stomach. Try eating a piece of fruit before going to any social gathering where you know there will be carb-loaded, processed snacks. You'll be amazed how much a juicy, sweet piece of fruit cuts your craving for salty, stale chips splashed with beer.

4. **COUNT TO YOUR AGE BEFORE YOU "CHEAT."** Anytime you find you are about to eat something that would be classified as "unhealthy," take the time to count to your age. Much of this sort of eating is impulsive and you don't actually take the time to think about whether you want to eat the item or not. You just cram it in and think nothing of it—until it creeps up onto your butt. If you still want to have a bite after your countdown, feel free: you've made a conscious decision to indulge, not a thoughtless gobble.

5. **AVOID EATING WITHIN TWO HOURS OF SLEEPING.** Eating right before you go to bed is a problem for two reasons. The first is that you don't have any opportunity to burn off the calories you've eaten before sleeping, so they are absorbed into your blood and transported around your body, where they are eventually stored as fat. The second problem is that, while you may be able to fall asleep right away, the digestive processes

going on in your stomach will require your brain to be partly awake, making your sleep much less restful and deep.

In the next chapter, we'll talk about how to navigate all the options you have for where and how to eat in college, and the logistics of eating economically and conveniently, without sacrificing good nutrition.

STEP 4

GET
A GRIP

*Where and How to Eat
Responsibly at College*

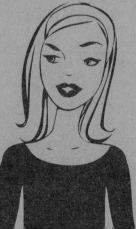

" I distinctly remember my first day at college as being one filled with stress—from the moving-in process, to long lines at registration, to being just plain hungry. I honestly could not find the dining hall until the third day of school."

—JESSICA, 19

A T FIRST, YOU might be overwhelmed with the food options available in the college dining hall: a hot bar with meats and vegetarian meal options (such as tofu scrambles and vegetable medleys); a salad bar; a grill with burgers, teriyaki bowls, grilled chicken breast, grilled cheeses, veggie burgers; a cereal stand; bread box; and every drink imaginable, from guava nectar to chocolate milk—oh, and my personal favorite, a soft-serve ice cream machine. I was so excited at the beginning of my freshman year, I loaded my tray up high with a bit of everything. And this was *after* I'd made my resolution to eat healthfully. There's something about an open buffet that wreaks havoc on any good eating resolutions.

While at first I would be balancing three different plates overloaded with food, I eventually realized that the cafeteria menu repeated itself. It dawned on me that it was not my last chance to have a grilled cheese if I didn't eat one that day. I began to adjust my eating habits so that I wasn't consuming half my body weight in food at every meal. I started going to the hot bar only at lunch, and having just a salad and a grilled chicken breast with cheese at dinner. I began making my own salad dressing with ingredients in the cafeteria: olive oil, balsamic vinegar, a dash of soy sauce, and a teaspoon of mustard whisked in a bowl with my spoon. That way, I wasn't getting all the sugars normally included in bottled dressings—and my version tasted better. I stopped drinking the concentrated fruit juices straight in favor of water, or water with some fruit juice. Sometimes I really just wanted a simple bowl of pasta, or the pizza that was the special of the evening, so I let myself have those things, but they were not regular fixtures on my dinner plate.

Dining hall food does get tedious, especially since there's only so much variation you can work into mass-produced meals. Happily, you'll probably have a lot of options when deciding where to eat at college, on campus or off.

In addition to our cafeteria, for instance, we also have a campus center that offers sushi, fresh fruit, pizza, frozen yogurt, sandwiches, salads, yogurt, hard-boiled eggs, and various beverages until 2 a.m. There's a convenience store and twenty-four-hour university store that offer the usual slew of packaged goods, including cereals, chips, candy, soda, ice cream, and frozen meals. Our university store even stocks foods from various shops in town, so I can have the tuna salad from the local deli day or night without even having to leave campus (albeit, for a higher price). If I'm eating at regular hours of the day, my college town has tons of restaurants, ranging from Indian to Japanese, and Italian to Korean. There's also a good supermarket within walking distance if I want to get groceries and make my own meals, which I do about twice a week, and a weekly on-campus farmer's market.

Your college town will most likely have similar eating venues, whether you go to school in a city where restaurants abound, or in a small town that thrives on the patronage of the student body. The point is: you can eat almost anything you want while away at school if you know where to look for it.

Of course, all these venues offer healthy and not-so-healthy options, and it's sometimes difficult to tell the difference. For instance, some restaurants and delis like to pretend that wraps are better for you than regular sandwiches because there is "less bread." This is a myth. A tortilla wrap is actually a much more condensed form of carbohydrates (usually simple carbohydrates) than regular bread and has about twice as many calories as two pieces of whole grain bread. Misinformation like this can cause even well-intentioned eaters to go off track; knowing exactly who your food friends and foes are—in the cafeteria, university store, dorm room, restaurant, and fast food establishment—will make it easier for you to beat the odds.

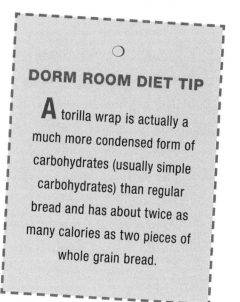

DORM ROOM DIET TIP

A torilla wrap is actually a much more condensed form of carbohydrates (usually simple carbohydrates) than regular bread and has about twice as many calories as two pieces of whole grain bread.

TIME, MONEY, AND STORAGE: IT'S ALL ABOUT BUDGETING

With the vast array of places to eat from which you can choose, you'll need to manage three things carefully: your time, your money, and your storage space. In order to establish a healthy eating regimen, it is essential to know the amount of time you have to eat, the amount of money you have to last you for the rest of the month, and how much of the fridge space is not taken over by your roommate's avocado face cream. All three concerns require budgeting.

Time

The first step, of course, is to determine your class schedule. After you've established when your windows of time are for meals, you can plan ahead to be sure you get something quick and healthful—at the very least, something from the grab-and-go list in Step 3. "Not enough time" is never a valid excuse for not eating breakfast. Everybody's busy these days, and with society so focused on saving time, new portable meals pop up every five seconds. You can try yogurt with a portable granola pouch, or a portable cup of just-add-water oatmeal. Whether you grab a piece of fruit and a low-fat yogurt on your way out the door, or take the extra minute to spread a thin layer of peanut butter on a piece of bread, eating on the go is easy. If you know you have a tendency to hit the snooze button a few times before rolling out of bed, put an apple in your bag the night before. (Don't try this with a banana, though; I once had to buy a new psychology text because I'd forgotten how responsible I'd been.)

If you happen to be an early riser, going to the cafeteria for breakfast is actually quite peaceful and relaxing, and you can get some heartier breakfast items like an omelet (opt for egg white, if you want to cut out the fat and cholesterol of the yolks). Also, knowing your schedule throughout the day will help you plan snacks so that you're eating something, even if it's just a handful of nuts, every two to four hours. That way, you won't be famished before any meal and will be less likely to overeat. You should try to head to dinner on the late side, around seven o'clock, since the lines will probably be shorter around that time and you won't be starving again by nine. Late-night eating is one of our chief foes, since there are few options to choose from if you haven't planned ahead and your body doesn't have the time to use up the calories you consumed before climbing into bed. But remember, try not to eat less than two hours before bed.

Money

If you're on the school eating plan, which many freshmen and sophomores are required to be, most of your food budget has been prepaid. And it's a good idea, since eating at the cafeteria can save you money, big time. Most schools partially subsidize cafeteria meals, so you can get a full, balanced meal for around five bucks. That's hard to beat. Of course, cafeteria food gets boring, and eating out once in a while is part of the experience of being at college. Going out to a meal is a social activity, a break from all the studying, a chance to visit a hot spot in town. Budgeting some cash to cover that occasional night out with the roomies or birthday dinner with a friend is crucial. You'll need to allocate food money by week, or even by day, to make sure that you are never left with an empty wallet.

Depending on how much money your parents are generous enough to give you monthly—or how much you are earning on your own through a part-time job—your budget for occasional eating out will vary. Say you have $200 a month for extra charges, outside of books and other supplies. That divides into about $50 per week, or about $7 a day. So, if you eat at the cafeteria for four of the seven days in a week, that means that you have $28 extra dollars for spending on the weekend, when it's more likely that you and your friends will get together for a splurge dinner or drinks. That goes fast. If you're stopping by Starbucks for a double latte every morning, keep in mind that you may be spending up to half of your daily cash allotment for that little eye opener. When you break it down this way, you realize that you really have to stick to your budget to get by.

Budgeting your allowance becomes even more important when you are trying to eat healthily, as these food options can sometimes prove to be more expensive than their fatty and fried counterparts. Of course, you can still make healthy eating choices on a limited budget. For instance, ordering just a healthy entrée instead of an appetizer and entrée could cut down on big spending, as well as calories. And the type of food you choose is important, too. I talked earlier about the price difference between pizza and sushi. While this is one scenario where enjoying the healthier sushi could mean having to dip a bit deeper into your slush fund, that doesn't mean that you should choose pizza instead. Sushi is generally a quick, highly nutritious, fairly accessible treat that you can enjoy on a special occasion. So you won't get to eat out as often if you're tight on cash from a few sushi nights, but your body will thank you for it. And there are even a few scenarios where eating well can actually *save* you money. For instance, rather than splurging twenty bucks on soda, popcorn, and candy at the movies, spend around $2 on a bottle of water and an apple before you get to the theater. Cut out calories and cut out cost. Perfect!

When it comes to grocery shopping, be sure to spend your money wisely. You can scavenge a lot of the basics from the cafeteria—salad items, vegetables, some hard fruits, even whole grain breads and cereals. Try to narrow your supermarket purchases to those health food items that aren't available on campus (like a special tofu preparation or high-fiber cereal). Also, while I am a berry fiend, I try to limit myself to a box or so a week because they can be very expensive—especially if you're buying them during the winter months when getting them to the Northeast United States, for instance, requires a whole lot of shipping costs or special growing conditions—and they don't keep very well. Only buy what you can eat in the next three days or so, and make multiple trips to the supermarket if need be. If it's within walking distance, this is a great way to score some extra exercise time as well. Lugging your groceries home definitely counts as a weight-bearing activity that helps burn calories and build lean muscle and bone mass. And remember, the beauty of college towns is that they're designed for students, many of whom are in the same financial boat, so there are plenty of eateries that offer a decent meal at prices that won't leave you washing dishes to pay for it. "Student specials" are nice perks if you can find them. Just as when you indulge in an unhealthy treat, going out to eat is something to be savored, and maybe even saved for special occasions only.

Storage

You'll have to negotiate with your roommate how you'll allocate fridge and storage space. It might be wise to invest in separate storage spaces if she's a real pain in the butt about not having your meat next to her vegan specialties. In any case, the fridge space in your room or hall will be limited, so you should look into purchasing things that don't need refrigeration (such as nuts, dried fruit, fruit leathers, popcorn, peanut butter, and cereal bars), and stay away from things that could rot on a hot night. Certain fresh fruits and vegetables can be pretty temperamental, not to mention expensive. Blueberries, for instance, are absolutely wonderful for you, but not if you're throwing out a moldy box of them at the end of the week because you forgot they were in the fridge. Not to mention the $3.49 that could have gone toward your weekend excursions going down the tube.

My roommates and I found that most of our fridge space was taken up with soda cans and bottles of water, leaving very little room for the leftovers and groceries that each of us brought home. My suggestion is that you designate a corner of your bookshelf as a snack corner and keep the nonperishables there. Make sure that you don't keep too many goodies on hand, though, or the temptation to snack on automatic pilot could become overwhelming. We'll talk more about eating while studying in Step 5, but be aware that having food too near your desk or workplace is never good: bored minds (and eyes) wander and food should not be in your line of vision. For the big stuff that needs storage (such as large cartons of milk, eggs, or lettuce), you can usually find a communal fridge in the dorm kitchen—a great place to cook simple meals, too. Just make sure you label anything you leave there, or you might find that Sticky Fingers in the room next to you made off with what was supposed to be tomorrow's breakfast.

Now that you're an expert on time, money, and storage issues, let's go find something healthy to eat!

THE CAFETERIA:
ONE-STOP SHOPPING

The cafeteria, you'll find, is truly a lifesaver. You have a huge variety of food from which to choose, so there is no excuse to eat poorly. You won't have to worry about missing out on your favorite entrée, since the cafeteria will usually repeat its menu several times throughout the year. Therefore, you know that if you choose to be good and refuse the mac-and-cheese today because you already had something less than nutritious earlier, you will have the chance to eat that dish later on in the month—maybe even that week. With such an array of food options available to you, you can be confident that you'll never go hungry, so there's no reason to stock up on extra calories. Also, there are often healthy eating initiatives on college campuses, usually student-headed, and the response has been tremendous. For instance, cafeterias across the country are now required to have vegetarian options available at every meal.

And here's the best part: you don't have to do any dishes, help prepare anything, or deal with any of the leftovers. (Many schools, however, do offer positions in cafeteria services, if you're looking to be paid.) For around five bucks you get to choose from salad, a hot meal bar, maybe even a grill. And because of the consistency of certain items (like the salad bar) and the variety of other sections (the hot meal bar will change its entrées for every meal), you can really get yourself into a good, healthful eating pattern without getting bored too quickly.

Of course, you'll probably be surrounded by an abundance of highly processed, highly fattening food, as well. The urge to eat these items becomes more pronounced when you see them every day and everyone around

DORM ROOM DIET TIP

Everything is about balance and nothing is off limits. If you overindulge today, eat healthfully tomorrow and the next day. Experts agree that the important thing is calorie intake over several days, not just one meal.

you seems to be enjoying them. Learning to pace yourself is the key to avoiding any serious weight gain, whether you're a freshman or a senior. The best way to do this without feeling deprived is to remember that everything is about balance and nothing is off limits. If you overindulge today, eat healthfully tomorrow and the next day. Experts agree that the important thing is calorie intake over several days, not just one meal. So don't be too hard on yourself if today was especially trying on your waistband; just get back on track tomorrow. A word of caution, though: if you eat poorly one day and healthfully the next, day after day, you'll be thwarting your efforts to get healthy and lose weight. If you are trying to drop pounds, don't eat the wrong stuff every other day and expect to be successful.

Here's what you need to know about cafeteria eating.

Your friends:

➤ Fresh fruits

➤ Fresh veggies

➤ Whole grain cereals (Total, All-Bran, Raisin Bran, Cheerios) and breads

➤ Low-fat cheese and milk

➤ Eggs (not fried)

➤ Grilled, baked, broiled, stir-fried, pan-seared anything

➤ Low-sugar, low-calorie items

Watch out, by the way, for the "low fat" head fake. Foods that you would normally assume to be high in fat, sugar, and calories but that for some reason aren't (for example, nonfat ice cream) are probably not very good for you. The manufacturers have to put something in there to replace the fat, so either you get lots of extra sugar or salt, or you get an artificial creation that your body can't digest and may cause certain types of cancers and diseases. For added incentive, see our discussion of artificial sweeteners in Step 3 if you're wondering why you really don't want them in your body. As a rule of thumb, go for naturally sweet items, like fruit, or find ways to get your sugar fix without overloading—a piece of chocolate rather than the whole bar, for instance. When you want to sweeten a drink, use sugar but dissolve it in warm water first. Dissolving it beforehand will cut down on the amount of sugar you need to achieve the desired sweetness. (You can also try a plant-derived cane sugar substitute, such as agave nectar, a cactus juice that tastes just like sugar and comes in liquid form, so you don't have to do the mixing.) The most common fat substitute, as you'll see when you

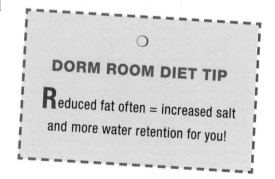

DORM ROOM DIET TIP

Reduced fat often = increased salt and more water retention for you!

look at the nutrition facts label of any diet/low-fat cookie carton, is sodium, or salt. While most teenagers don't really need to worry about having too much salt, it does make you retain water, which leads to bloating.

Your foes:

➤ Stewed or jellied fruits (which have tons of sugar)

➤ Sugary cereals

➤ High-sugar fruit and soda drinks

➤ Full-fat cheese, milk

➤ Fried anything

➤ Cheesy, creamy sauces

➤ Full-fat, high-sugar items (ice cream, cookies, brownies, cakes)

➤ Simple carbohydrates (rice, crackers, bagels—except for the whole grain varieties)

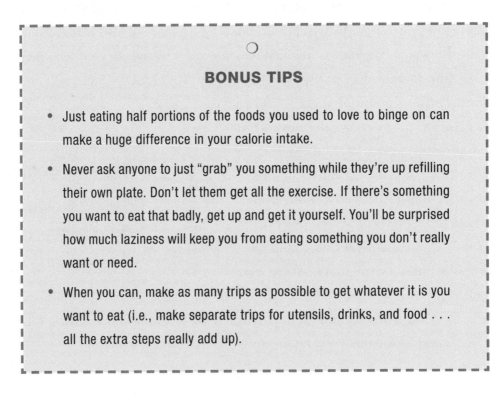

BONUS TIPS

• Just eating half portions of the foods you used to love to binge on can make a huge difference in your calorie intake.

• Never ask anyone to just "grab" you something while they're up refilling their own plate. Don't let them get all the exercise. If there's something you want to eat that badly, get up and get it yourself. You'll be surprised how much laziness will keep you from eating something you don't really want or need.

• When you can, make as many trips as possible to get whatever it is you want to eat (i.e., make separate trips for utensils, drinks, and food . . . all the extra steps really add up).

Again, I can't stress enough the importance of balance. I am not talking about a total ban on these "foes," but I'm not talking about an equal distribution between the unhealthful options and the healthful ones, either—at least not if you are trying to lose weight. Especially for those of you who are trying to get healthy, not just skinny, avoid the unhealthful options whenever you can.

IN YOUR DORM

Most dormitories will have limited space to store healthful foods and a high concentration of packaged, sugary foods on site. This may be especially true if you are not relying on your own shopping skills, but are sharing your roommates' food preferences. In order to stick to your healthy lifestyle, you've got to get creative.

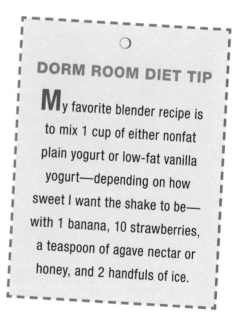

DORM ROOM DIET TIP

My favorite blender recipe is to mix 1 cup of either nonfat plain yogurt or low-fat vanilla yogurt—depending on how sweet I want the shake to be—with 1 banana, 10 strawberries, a teaspoon of agave nectar or honey, and 2 handfuls of ice.

In a highly controlled, scientific study I conducted my freshman year, it became evident that I would much rather chow down a chocolate bar than eat a carton of strawberries. By microwaving the chocolate bar and dipping the strawberries into the melted chocolate, however, not only did I eat just a quarter of the chocolate bar, but I found myself full after this not-so-evil snack. The chocolate bar alone would have left me hungry for more, because it contains no fiber to counterbalance the huge sugar intake, and the resulting insulin spike; with strawberries, you get all the fleshy, fibrous goodness to slow the insulin release. I still got the taste of chocolate, but I found I needed less than I thought I did to satisfy my craving—a striking revelation! You won't be able to avoid junk food the whole time you're in college. You will just need to find innovative ways to balance your psyche's needs for "bad" stuff with your body's need for the "good" stuff.

Your friends:

➤ Fresh fruits (especially with some unsweetened peanut butter, or lemon juice and 1/2 teaspoon of sugar to spice things up)

➤ Nuts

➤ Veggies (baby carrots are accessible, easy to store, and great for when you need that crunch)

➤ Seltzer with a splash of fruit juice

➤ Diet, low-sugar, low-fat, low-carb, low-cal anything— not so healthy, but less fattening than their regular alternatives

Your foes:

➤ Highly processed foods (chips, candy, etc.)

➤ Sugary foods and drinks (surprised?)

➤ Anything made primarily from white flour (muffins, cookies, pastry)

○
BONUS TIPS

- As a last resort, just have small portions of the evil stuff. Serve yourself in a small attractive dish, preferably glass or ceramic, so you feel satisfied, not deprived. (Standing in front of a refrigerator digging a spoon into a half-gallon of ice cream just makes you feel fat and slovenly.) And don't go back for seconds.

- Bring your own food or eat before you join the party.

- Be inventive. Like my chocolate-dipped strawberry example, find ways to enjoy the foods you can't live without, but do so in either smaller portions, or combined with some other food that will make it easier for you to say you're already full and mean it. Almost any fruit can be dipped in melted chocolate. You can also try cut-up fruit with lemon juice and a little sugar . . . it adds zest to the plain fruit but without adding that many more calories, plus the lemon juice acts as an appetite suppressant.

- I know you'll have a blender on hand, so give it a rest from margarita making and whip up a fruit, low-fat yogurt, and honey smoothie. It's a great snack or small meal, loaded with fiber, calcium, vitamin D, and enzymes . . . all packed into a sweet and delicious mix.

IN RESTAURANTS

Everyone loves going out to a nice dinner. Until it's time to order and you're torn between getting your favorite, fettuccine Alfredo, and knowing that you should really stick to a nice piece of grilled fish. To make matters worse, guess which one is more expensive? The battle wages in your head: heavy, creamy pasta or lean, flavorful fish? You decide which wins out. Thankfully, you now know just how fattening the fettuccine is, with its simple carbohydrate pasta coupled with heavy cream sauce; you also know about the wonderful omega fats and protein in the fish. Easy decision, right? Sometimes . . .

Eating out at restaurants is a lot like eating in the cafeteria, because you have a huge selection of options, some healthy and some not. Learning to eat healthfully in general can ease the stress of eating-out decisions: even though you might like the idea of a rich, cheesy pasta dinner, you know how bad it is for you in the long run. Sometimes you're willing to take the risk, but most of the time you should give your body a break and go with some premium fuel. Take advantage of the fact that the restaurant's chefs know how to prepare vegetables, fish, and other healthy options that are much better than the varieties you'll be able to find in your dorm or cafeteria.

Your friends:

- ➤ Complex carbohydrates
- ➤ Salad with olive oil and lemon/vinegar
- ➤ Vegetables or fruits
- ➤ Fish and other lean proteins, baked, broiled, pan-seared, or grilled
- ➤ Eggs, nonfried

Your foes:

- ➤ Fried preparations of anything

- ➤ Cheesy, fatty sauces or fruit glazes

- ➤ Simple carbohydrates

- ➤ Salads with creamy dressings

- ➤ Sugary drinks (lemonade, sweetened iced tea, etc.)

○

BONUS TIPS

- If you must have pasta, opt for the whole wheat preparations. If there are none on the menu, go for regular pasta with a light tomato sauce. Marinara, primavera, or other sauces that are basically just tomatoes, vegetables, olive oil, and herbs are your best bet.

- Ask the waiter to bring whole wheat or whole grain bread if it is available and put no butter on it, only olive oil. Have a piece of bread dipped in olive oil before the meal to curb your hunger.

- Have a small piece of fruit before going out to dinner. This will take the edge off your hunger and make you less likely to overeat.

FAST FOOD RATION

Fast food burger chains are potential minefields for the healthy eater. Only recently are healthy options being introduced to these venues, and even these are a far cry from ideal. If a road trip with friends finds you on the drive-thru line or making a pit stop, you should be prepared. This is an especially important time to remember that cutting portions—small fries instead of large, junior-size burger rather than the Daddy—can make a huge difference. There are also those newly added healthy menu options, such as salads, whole grain premium sandwiches, and grilled chicken.

The same goes for gas station convenience store visits. An entire establishment dedicated to the "Cookies, Candy, Chips" section of the grocery store, this could be the healthy eater's worst foe. I know very few people who, after several hours in the car, can resist the temptation to dive into a sweet or salty snack.

> ## FAST FOOD TIPS
>
> 1. Be wary of prepackaged dressings—they're often loaded with sugars and extra calories. Always go for just oil and vinegar when you can.
>
> 2. Use marinara sauce or organic ketchup instead of other sauces whenever possible—they have little or no fat and potentially less sugar.
>
> 3. Stay away from anything fried: that includes the croutons on your salad.

It may be because most people are not aware of the new healthful options now available in most gas stations, such as soy nuts, dried fruit and nuts, or even fresh fruit in some areas. In any case, no fast food establishment should be entered without extreme caution and a steely resolve to avoid certain items.

Your friends:

- ➤ Protein, preferably lean (chicken breast, hamburger, fish sandwich, not fried)

- ➤ Small portions of anything

- ➤ Salads (fast food salads are improving, and at some you can even choose low-fat Ranch or Italian, rather than fatty French—hey, it's a start)

- ➤ Yogurt (instead of ice cream, apple pies, or other sweets)

- ➤ Sandwiches on whole grain breads (without tons of mayo—go for low-fat if you can)

- ➤ Fruit salad

- ➤ Nuts

- ➤ Water or sports drinks before soda

Your foes:

- ➤ Fried anything

- ➤ Anything with full-fat dairy (cheeseburger, cheese fries, ice cream, creamy soup)

- ➤ Sugary drinks and sodas

- ➤ Sugary dressings

Now you know what to eat at college. You know how and when and where to eat, too. That was the easy stuff. You're about to learn just how scary college can be. Get ready for our next step: The Five Danger Zones.

○

BONUS TIPS

- Opt for those low-fat dressings, and use sparingly as they probably have a lot of sugar and salt to compensate for less fat.

- Whenever you can, go for grilled. "Extra crispy" just means more bread and more oil.

- Try to fit in vegetables and protein whenever possible (like a veggie bean burrito).

- Always ask for low-fat or nonfat dairy products.

- Eat raw fruits and veggies whenever available.

- If you must eat at a fast food restaurant, go for a salad. If you can't get a salad (or don't want to), get the leanest meat you can find (skinless poultry or fish, preferably) or a veggie burger. If you don't want either of those, go for the hamburger, but nix the cheese and special sauce. And, finally, if you absolutely must have these accoutrements, go for the smallest size available. Keep in mind, that one 4-ounce burger (no bun, mayo, or special sauce included) is 360 calories, the same as the calorie count in four veggie burgers.

- Read the book *Fast Food Nation* by Eric Schlosser. You might never set foot in a fast food restaurant again. (Yeah, it's that convincing.)

STEP 5

GET PREPARED

*The Five Danger Zones
and How to Survive Them*

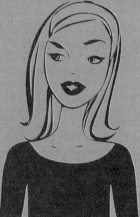

"It was about 10 p.m. the night before my biology final and I still had four chapters to go through—I knew it was going to be a long night. So I ran to the university store to grab a diet soda and some coffee. While I was there, I figured I should also probably grab a few snacks to keep me going. Of course, I didn't opt for the carrot-and-celery-stick combo. By the time I checked out, I was laden down with tortilla chips, salsa, chocolate chip cookies, and a few bags of gummy bears—plus the soda and coffee. I paced myself over the next five hours, but by the time I crawled into bed at 3 a.m. I was exhausted and feeling sick from having eaten everything."

—JENNA, 20

JUST BECAUSE YOU can most likely find anything you want to eat on or around your college campus, it doesn't mean that an abundance of unhealthy options won't be there to sidetrack you along the way. Of course, you could simply try to avoid any event or situation on campus that might be accompanied by cookies, chips, pizza, beer, fries, and candy. You could have also stayed in your parents' house in Ohio.

In this chapter I want to give you a heads-up on the five most common sinkholes of unhealthy eating that you'll encounter during your college years. There is nothing quite so hard as resisting the urge to dive into that open bag of tortilla chips as you're pulling another all-nighter, watching the last basketball quarter, holding up the wall at a party, viewing the season finale of your fave TV show, or engaging in a life-defining discussion with your roommate. Deciding to eat something because you want to and are willing to allow yourself a small treat is one thing. Eating nutritionally devoid, fattening foods because you are trying to procrastinate, socialize, or are bored, and because "everybody else is doing it," is another. When you find yourself eating when you're not really hungry and without tasting what's in your mouth, you're eating for distraction. You've entered a danger zone.

Remember that allowing yourself to eat something naughty *sometimes* (in moderation) is what makes the Dorm Room Diet fun and easy to stick with. Feeling continually deprived of what you crave will likely send you right back to unhealthy eating habits. To find out how to make indulgence work for you, rather than against you, read on.

HOW TO CHEAT IN MODERATION: INDULGING FOR A GOOD CAUSE

If you eat something unhealthy, it should fuel your resolve to eat better in the future, not send you spiraling into a vortex of guilt that can only be stopped by eating the rest of the box of cookies, doughnuts, or whatever else you'd chosen to nibble on. Unfortunately, this is not always the way our psyches work. Along with the negative feelings we have about diets in general, we have attached negative feelings to enjoying food that we know isn't healthful.

Because so many diets prescribe very strict rules, going off for even a tiny treat can be disastrous. (For example, on Atkins, you get all your energy from the tremendous amount of fat and protein you consume; if you eat even the tiniest morsel of carbohydrate, all the fat stops being used for fuel and settles around your middle instead.) Because about 60 percent of Americans are on a diet at any given time, a majority of us are perpetually worried about eating what we want for fear of sabotaging our weight-loss efforts. Even worse, once we

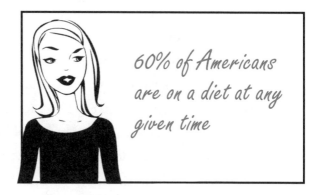

60% of Americans are on a diet at any given time

cheat—even a little bit—we start rationalizing: "Well, I've already been bad today, so it's okay to gorge on anything I want. I'll start fresh tomorrow."

Let's say Rebecca is trying to eat healthfully, but somehow she finds herself face-to-face with a plate of warm chocolate chip cookies. Now, Rebecca is no glutton, but she reasons that if she's going to give in to one cookie, it's probably smart to get the craving for cookies out of her system by eating four or five more, since, after this binge is over, she won't be having any more of these babies for at least a lifetime. Rebecca was probably satisfied after that first cookie, and she'd consumed only about 100 calories at that point. Her self-imposed punishment—overeating junk food really is punishment, because it makes you suffer by thwarting all your hard work to lose weight and get healthy—of eating five more cookies, however, brings her calorie intake to 600 big ones. Even worse, it's unlikely that this binge will stop her from eating another cookie (or five) the next time a steaming plate is brought before her.

When Marlow is presented with the same plate of cookies, she allows herself to enjoy the first cookie, savoring its gooey goodness to the max. But she realizes that every cookie after that will taste the same. She won't get any more satisfaction from the next one, so she quits while she's ahead. Marlow *chooses* not to feel guilty for enjoying a special treat, feels *satisfied* with one cookie, and does not feel the need to punish herself. By cheating in moderation, she doesn't have to worry when, on another night a week later, she wants to have one more cookie.

Most of us don't take the time to enjoy the small indulgences we allow ourselves because we know we "shouldn't" be eating something so deliciously bad. Better that we cram it down our throats quickly without thinking. But where does that leave us? Stuffed and bloated on cookies we didn't even enjoy. Going cold turkey and never allowing ourselves any treats isn't the perfect solution either, because this leaves you feeling deprived and sorry for yourself, making fulfillment of your goals highly improbable. Part of being able to eat in moderation is knowing that you will have the opportunity to eat that thing again; there's no need to stockpile now. The business of eating healthfully is a marathon, not a sprint.

When you do cheat, make it worthwhile. Choose your indulgences carefully. A small slice of that exquisite cake at your best friend's birthday party is probably worth it; yesterday's leftover bagels—with extra butter to make up for the staleness—is not. Once again, with the Dorm Room Diet nothing's off limits and everything is in bounds. This freedom should make the lure of eating an unhealthy item less appealing. But, if you do choose to eat it, eat slowly and savor every bite—don't gobble it down expecting to have another one immediately afterward. If you find that even after slowly enjoying the first treat you can't resist having another, do your age countdown as we discussed in Step 3 (see page 83). If that doesn't work, simply remove yourself from the temptation; even moving to another part of the table (far from the offending plate of cookies) may be enough to keep you from making a decision you'll regret.

WORTH CHEATING FOR . . .

A small slice of birthday cake

Homemade brownies or cookies

Dessert after a nice dinner out with friends or family

Truly spectacular sweets that you are willing to travel for, like the Magnolia Bakery cupcakes my roommate and I make road trips to New York City for

Grilled cheese, which you've haven't had in weeks

NOT WORTH CHEATING FOR . . .

A piece of birthday cake in a flavor you know you hate

Cafeteria or store-bought cookies or brownies

Dessert every time you eat a meal

A mediocre pastry at a social event

Grilled cheese, when you just had it yesterday

DANGER ZONE #1: MAKING THE DEADLINE—STUDYING FOR TESTS AND WRITING PAPERS

You go to college to enrich your mind and broaden your knowledge, so classes are a top priority. Because few schools are progressive enough to do away with grades, you'll most likely be taking some tests and writing some graded papers during your time at college. Studying or writing for a deadline anytime is stressful, but, if you're anything like me, procrastination will ensure that most of your work is done right before the due date in long stretches extending into the wee hours of the morning. (I do not recommend this, by the way!) For me, the material seems especially boring at these times and I am easily distracted by the images of sleep and food that keep wandering through my head. Sleep is not an option, so pick-me-up snacks become a must. But what to eat at 2 a.m. when everything but the university store is closed? Most likely, the options are limited to simple carbohydrates if you are not prepared for this sort of situation.

Studying for tests and writing papers is a danger zone because:

1. You're sitting still for a long period of time and get restless.

2. You're under stress and might make hasty decisions about what to eat.

3. You don't have time to forage for good, healthy food.

4. You typically only have highly processed food available on hand.

5. You want food and beverages that will help you stay awake and alert.

The following tips will help you
avoid disaster:

1. **PREPARE FOR A LONG NIGHT BY KEEPING THESE
   SNACKS ON HAND:**

   ➤ baby carrots

   ➤ almonds

   ➤ 1 grapefruit

   ➤ 1 apple

   ➤ 1 pear

   ➤ 2 small handfuls of semisweet chocolate chips

   ➤ 1 bag of rice cakes or soy crisps, flavored or not

All of these items are easy to find on or around campus, they're cheap, and they'll help to keep you from turning to less healthy options. The baby carrots are great because they fulfill that desire for crunch that would otherwise come from pretzels or another crisp, salty snack. Grapefruit is a natural appetite suppressant and, because it takes a little time to peel and eat, it gives you a nice break from studying, with the added benefit of lots of vitamin C to keep you alert. The apple and pear are two low-sugar fruits that are easy to store and have when you're in the middle of a study spree. And the bag of semisweet chocolate chips is to satisfy your craving for sweet,

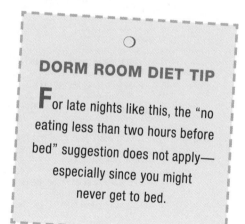

DORM ROOM DIET TIP

For late nights like this, the "no eating less than two hours before bed" suggestion does not apply—especially since you might never get to bed.

DORM ROOM DIET TIP

When studying late, at the end of the first hour, have a small handful of almonds or some baby carrots. At the end of the second hour, have a grapefruit, apple, or pear. At the end of the third hour, you can have a small handful of semisweet chocolate chips or some soy crisps. Keep going in this pattern for as long as you are studying and feel like you want a little something to munch on.

fatty foods that will increase as the study hours wear on. Because they are semisweet, they have less sugar than milk chocolate, so a small handful of them contains only about 100 calories. The rice cakes or soy crisps are salty-crunchy craving fixers, with very few calories and little to no sugar. Also, the soy crisps have very few carbs and, on average, about 7 grams of protein per serving.

2. EMERGEN-C PACKETS ARE EFFERVESCENT, SINGLE-SERVING PACKETS OF ENERGY.
All you need to do is dump a packet into a glass of water and you have an incredibly energizing drink ready to go. Keep a bottle of this stuff next to you while you study to keep you hydrated and awake. There are about ten flavors to choose from. A box of sixty packets costs about $20 and they keep forever, so you won't have to worry about them going bad. Much better for you than the caffeine in soda, tea, or coffee, too, since they deliver energy through a high dose of vitamin C and other vitamins and minerals.

3. GIVE YOURSELF SCHEDULED BREAKS DURING WHICH YOU'VE ALREADY PLANNED WHAT TO EAT.
You'll be more productive during your study time because there's a reward at the end of each interval. So, for instance,

WHY IS LATE-NIGHT
SIMPLE CARB LOADING SO BAD

Any simple carbs that you eat late at night will most likely end up as fat (since you won't be doing much exercising while you sleep), and sleeping on a full stomach invariably leaves you starving in the morning, and not for yogurt and some fruit. You want carbs! This is because your bloodstream goes from being packed with sugar (glucose quickly broken down from the simple carbs) to having almost none at all (the glucose you don't use as fuel is stored in the muscles as glycogen), and is looking to replenish. If you eat a more fibrous pre-bedtime snack, the process of breaking down the sugars takes a good deal longer, providing a slow release of glucose into the bloodstream. This way, by the time you get up in the morning, there is still sugar circulating in your blood.

Morning carb binges (pancakes, waffles, bagels, and sweetened, refined cereals) set you up for a day of carb cravings, most likely leading to meals with few nutrients and high sugar and fat content. That simple carb loading begets more simple carb loading—rather than satiating the craving—is an unfortunate fact of life. If you spike your bloodstream with an initial jolt of easy sugar, you will crave another hit all day—just like a junkie. Put that junkie in rehab by making sure you begin your day with a meal full of fiber, a little bit of fat, and some protein, rather than simple carbs. An omelet (egg whites only or not) with veggies and organic meat is a great option. You can throw a high-fiber fruit (like an apple) in there for good measure, too, or as a midmorning munch.

at the end of the first hour have a small handful of almonds or some baby carrots. At the end of the second hour, have a grapefruit, apple, or pear. At the end of the third hour, you can have a small handful of semisweet chocolate chips or some soy crisps. Keep going in this pattern for as long as you are studying and feel like you want a little something to munch on.

4. **INTERMITTENTLY TAKE BREAKS TO GO TO THE BATHROOM AND SPLASH WARM WATER FIVE TIMES AND THEN COOL WATER FIVE TIMES ONTO YOUR FACE.** Follow with a few clean, cool splashes on and into your eyes. This will not only wake you up and keep your eyes from getting dry and weary, but it will also clean any bacteria off your face from leaning on your hands while you're studying or touching your face absentmindedly, so you can avoid acne breakouts. You can also take a brisk walk or climb a few flights of stairs to get the blood circulating after a long sitting session.

DANGER ZONE #2: TAILGATING AND SPORTS EVENTS

During my sophomore year at Princeton, our football team beat Yale University for the first time in ten years. As part of the "big three" (Princeton, Harvard, Yale) rivalry, we were promised a huge bonfire if our team won against Harvard the following weekend.

There was a record-breaking turnout for the game, but an even larger one for the pregame tailgate parties. Each fraternity or sorority had its own setup, as did individual groups of friends, various campus clubs, and families who had come in for the big game. It was all great fun—the smell of the barbecue, the feeling of camaraderie, the thrill of competition in the air. But, as with any sporting event party worth its salt (literally), this tailgate involved carloads of potato chips, full-fat dips, simple carb buns for the burgers and hot dogs, and desserts of brownies, cookies, and ice cream—and, of course, lots and lots of beer. We spent the day watching other people exercise, and making bags of popcorn, six-foot hoagies, and candy bars disappear.

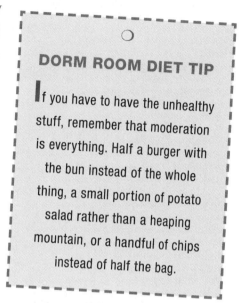

DORM ROOM DIET TIP

If you have to have the unhealthy stuff, remember that moderation is everything. Half a burger with the bun instead of the whole thing, a small portion of potato salad rather than a heaping mountain, or a handful of chips instead of half the bag.

It's always hard to avoid indulging when everyone around you is eating and drinking the same stuff and the game goes on for hours on end. Especially when the stakes are high, you can find yourself eating out of a range of emotions—from anticipation to boredom, celebration to commiseration. Unfortunately, Princeton lost to Harvard that day and we did not get a bonfire, or a postgame party. Who knows how long the bingeing would have continued if we'd had more to celebrate?

Tailgating and sports events are a danger zone because:

1. You want to take part with friends in an activity that is centered around eating, but the food options are mostly limited to unhealthful choices.

2. You are bored by the sports event you're watching and turn to food to pass the time.

3. You like to celebrate a point or victory for your team by eating.

4. You want to soothe your sorrow over a bad call or a loss with food.

The following tips will help you avoid disaster:

1. Have a bunless hamburger or hot dog.

2. Stay away from potato salad, creamy coleslaw, or anything else with a lot of mayonnaise and fat.

3. Offer to bring some dessert for the tailgate and bring a fruit salad, a healthy, satisfying palate cleanser for the end of the meal.

4. Stick to water or club soda (regular soda as a last resort) and peanuts at games, or pack an apple in your bag before you go.

5. Feel free to jeer at the other team and holler like a cheerleader when you want to celebrate your team's good work, but don't celebrate your team's success by sabotaging your own.

6. If you have to have the unhealthy stuff, remember that moderation is everything. Half a burger instead of the whole thing, a small portion of potato salad rather than a heaping mountain, or a handful of chips instead of half the bag.

7. Move around and get different views of the game from points around the stadium. That way, you're getting in some extra steps rather than sitting for three hours straight, so you can eat some of what you love and have something to do besides sitting and eating.

DANGER ZONE #3: PARTIES AND OTHER CAMPUS GATHERINGS

"I feel most self-conscious about trying to eat healthfully when I'm at a party. I mean, if I'm constantly thinking about how I can't eat the snacks that are there, I'm clearly not enjoying the party that much. And I'm usually really hungry by the time I get to a late-night party, so I'm staring at the food and not eating any of it, which is just awkward."

—RACHEL, 19

Room and hallway parties are a great way to meet your neighbors, bond with friends, and just celebrate in general. Parties are all about having fun and letting loose with pals. They should not be events that make you feel awkward or self-conscious, and they are especially not times when you should be consumed with thinking about food. Since you know that party fare consists largely of chips, pretzels, and chocolate everything, it's important that you prepare for party nights ahead of time. Eat a few snacks or a small meal before the party so you're not obsessing about *not* eating. Whatever you do, don't come to a party famished, or you'll casually end up downing a whole bowl of potato chips without even noticing, which won't make anyone more comfortable.

Campus gatherings, like club meetings or information hours, present another challenge: they can be really tedious and eating helps pass the time. Unfortunately, the platter of fatty cheeses and processed crackers normally provided don't really meet the healthy requirement, especially if they're replacing a meal and you'll need to eat a lot of them to feel satisfied. Bringing your own food, especially if you bring it only for yourself, can seem rude (and strange). To prepare for any food temptations you might encounter at these affairs, eat an apple or pear before you get going to stave off hunger so you are less likely to crave a lot of the bad stuff.

Parties are a danger zone because:

1. There is a lot of unhealthful food available.

2. You are distracted by talking and being with the other people, so you aren't conscious of what you are eating.

3. You can't acceptably bring your own food to a social gathering.

4. You eat to look busy or to do something with your hands.

5. You eat to feel like part of the group.

Follow these tips to avoid disaster:

1. Eat an apple or pear before you get to the party to put something in your stomach: it will keep you full and make you less likely to eat a lot of junk food at the party. You can also try a citrus fruit, like a grapefruit, which, in addition to the fiber it provides, acts as a natural appetite suppressant. Add a protein to your fruit/fiber to really get rid of any craving. Try unsweetened peanut butter, low-fat cheese, or hummus.

2. Position yourself away from the food table, so that the food is "out of sight, out of mind."

3. Arrive at the party chewing gum. It will keep your mouth moving (so you aren't tempted to eat), and your breath fresh, and may also increase your metabolism, in addition to thoroughly washing your teeth with extra saliva.

4. Keep a cup of water or a low-sugar beverage in hand at all times so your hands feel like they're doing something. Also, drinking lots of fluid will keep you feeling full so you aren't tempted to stock up on the snacks.

5. Think about how great you look at this party because you've been doing so well with the Dorm Room Diet, and how you want to look even better at the next one.

DANGER ZONE #4: WATCHING TV

My friends and I make time to watch TV together every night: *24* on Mondays, *House* on Tuesdays, *America's Next Top Model* on Wednesdays, *The O.C.* on Thursdays, and movie night on Fridays. We sometimes end up ordering in, even if some of us have already been to dinner before our show comes on. Commercial breaks provide the perfect opportunity to quickly stuff down some food.

Our constant sitting-and-eating routine was beginning to catch up with us, so we decided to watch TV in a different room each night. Since our campus is pretty large, this meant that everyone ended up walking at least a half-mile each night. Even this little bit helped. Not only did we burn a few extra calories but exercise also suppresses your appetite, so, by the time we got to the TV "host" room, we weren't so hungry for the takeout of the evening.

While you may find that you don't actually have much time to watch TV at school, the time you do spend in front of the tube can be very dangerous for your new healthy lifestyle. It's a sedentary, passive activity, so your mind easily wanders to the snacks sitting in the corner of the room. And it's usually done in a group, which makes it harder to resist temptations others are indulging in. If you do choose to have a snack, the fact that you are distracted by the television impairs your ability to enjoy the food, gauge how satisfied you are with the amount you've eaten, and know when to stop. Therefore, it's best to put whatever you are going to eat in an individual bowl, rather than to munch out of a bag or box, so you know exactly how much you've eaten. If you know that you're someone who works better within a structured environment, make a rule: eat only at a table, not on the couch or the floor, and only from your designated, individual-serving bowl.

Watching TV is a danger zone because:

1. You are not actively involved in doing anything, so your mind wanders, often settling on the desire to snack.

2. You will normally only have time to watch TV after dinner, which means that whatever calories you eat will not have much time to be burned off before you go to bed. And, because you've already had dinner, you're not eating out of hunger, you're eating out of boredom, which always spells danger.

3. You'll look for quick, convenient snacks, to avoid missing any of your show. This means you're probably eating highly processed carbohydrates out of a bag or a box, which means you won't know how much you've eaten (unless you eat the entire box, in

which case, I'm not sure you want to know how much you've eaten).

4. You want to go along with the crowd. If the groupthink says that ordering in is natural and necessary to enjoying television with friends, who are you to contradict?

In order to avoid disaster you can:

1. Drink a glass of water before you have anything to eat; a lot of times, we confuse thirst with hunger.

2. Chew gum.

3. Always try to have a piece of fruit rather than processed snacks, especially late at night. If plain fruit doesn't cut it, try some peanut butter or low-fat cheese with the fruit. You can also dip your fruit in chocolate and refrigerate it, so if you need a little chocolate, you can grab an already dipped piece of fruit in a hurry.

4. Keep a bag of semisweet chocolate chips around, so if you want a sweet fix you can take a small handful.

5. Try rice cakes or soy crisps before turning to more processed snacks; they come in a variety of flavors and the soy crisps even give you some protein without much fat.

> **DORM ROOM DIET TIP**
>
> **A**lways try to have a piece of fruit rather than processed snacks, especially late at night. If plain fruit doesn't cut it, try some peanut butter or low-fat cheese with the fruit. You can also dip your fruit in chocolate and refrigerate it, so if you need a little chocolate, you can grab an already dipped piece of fruit in a hurry.

6. If you really have to have something carbohydrate-based and processed, try separating snacks into bags of single-serving portions ahead of time, so you know how much you've eaten and won't be tempted to eat whatever amount "the claw" retrieves during its five dives into the box. Wheat Thins or Triscuits are good choices here, because they're baked (not fried) and made with whole grain.

DANGER ZONE #5: LATE-NIGHT TALKS

I mentioned earlier how college is a place to find yourself, and late-night talks with friends and roommates are part of this process. You're going through a lot of new experiences, a lot of stresses, and somehow the day doesn't seem complete until you've laid them all out and analyzed them to smithereens with the girls. Sometimes your thoughts seem most vivid and clear late at night when the dorm is quiet and the intimacy of sharing secrets seems heightened. I know I go into "overshare" mode whenever it's been a long day and I have my best friend trapped in the room next to mine. Once, I related an extremely detailed story about my debacle with a sociology professor whom I hated—a very sordid yarn of passive-aggressive attacks on my part and complete obliviousness on his—only to find she'd been asleep the whole time.

As nice as it is to talk about every-

> **DORM ROOM DIET TIP**
>
> Have some sparkling water with fruit juice as a sweet fix before you eat anything. The bubbles will fill you up and won't leave you feeling bloated from having carbs right before bed.

thing with friends, there are some not-so-nice aspects to this scenario. I found that whenever I got into these conversations, whether I was discovering who I am as a person, or just rehashing old gossip, food would somehow find its way into my mouth. I was happy to have someone to talk to, glad that we made progress in understanding each other and ourselves, or even upset when things didn't go my way if we happened to be arguing. All these factors made it easy to justify having a few chips *and* some ice cream *and* whatever else was lying around the room. Food, once again, seemed to accelerate the bonding process.

Late-Night Talks are a danger zone because:

1. You are enjoying bonding with your friends and aren't thinking about what goes into your mouth.

2. It's many hours since the cafeteria closed for dinner, and your body is starting to get hungry again.

3. It's late at night and you're getting tired, so you eat to stay awake.

4. Whatever you eat sits in your stomach while you sleep, making you sleep fitfully and possibly causing you to gain weight.

How to avoid disaster:

1. If you're in your own room having these chats, make sure that it is free of unhealthy temptations.

2. Have some sparkling water with fruit juice as a sweet fix before you eat anything. The bubbles will fill you up and won't leave you feeling bloated from having carbs right before bed.

3. Have some berries. They take time to eat, come in small pieces, and are sweet enough to sometimes remove the need to eat less healthful alternatives.

4. If you do succumb, make sure you know exactly how much unhealthy stuff you're eating by measuring it into a bowl. By all means avoid eating ice cream out of the carton, as spoonfuls quickly add up to pints, especially if you're sharing with friends.

AVOIDING ADDICTIVE FOODS

When eating with friends, avoid certain "addictive" foods. Addictive foods are those that increase your cravings for more of the same kind and those that give you a short-lived mood boost. Some examples of addictive food are candy, refined carbs, ice cream, and other whole-fat dairy items—pretty much the bad guys we've been dealing with throughout this book.

We turn to these foods for comfort when we're feeling sad, angry, depressed, or bored. More often than not, the long-term result of our quick-fix selection is weight gain, along with persistent feelings of sadness, anger, depression, or boredom. This is because we become addicted to the good feelings we get from eating our fix and become incapable of coping without it. Thus, we indulge more often and in larger quantities than is healthy or necessary. Depriving yourself of the food that seems so crucial at a particular moment in time, however, can leave you fixated on eating or not eating it, again diverting your attention from dealing with your feelings. What we often don't realize is that food cannot make us feel "good" permanently; we need to resolve the issue that made us unhappy in the first place.

Because it's very difficult to do a complete psychological makeover in an instant, it may take some time to wean yourself off any food crutch you might have. Depending on the strength of your willpower, you may be able to eat safely a very limited portion of your food of choice. For some, this small taste would open the floodgates of nutritional hell. For others, it might be just the thing to alleviate cravings. You know yourself best, so you'll have to gauge whether it is riskier to indulge or not.

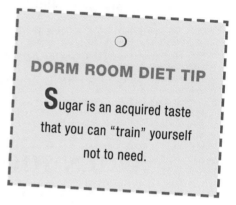

DORM ROOM DIET TIP

Sugar is an acquired taste that you can "train" yourself not to need.

Should you choose the drastic change option and observe total abstinence, there are other ways to boost your mood and cope with unhappy feelings without food. For starters, get out of the environment where the temptation is available. Exercise, especially exercise that requires you to focus your mind (such as yoga), not only relaxes the body, but also signals the brain to release endorphins, another one of our "happy" chemicals. The raised level of endorphins alleviates stress and tells your body that you don't have a care in the world, so there is no reason to be so uptight. Step 6 goes into the various workouts you can try, including conventional cardio, yoga, Pilates, and relaxing breathing exercises. You can't help but feel calm and energized after any thorough, aerobic workout. Of course, this exercise high will wear off in a few hours. But needing to do a repeat workout (as long as you don't overwork yourself) is a much healthier option than doing a repeat kitchen raid.

If exercising doesn't sound like a fair trade-off for giving up your doughnut-hole binges, try finding a healthier snack that satiates your cravings. For instance, *fruit leathers* are a great, sweet snack with one quarter the calories of a candy bar. Dried fruit and nuts or a teaspoon of peanut butter might do the trick. Experiment with healthy options. Pretend you're a caveman, and the genius who invented packaged candy bars hasn't yet graced the planet. No need to go out and hunt down a woolly mammoth; just find something that is naturally sweet, salty, or creamy. Remember that sugar is an acquired taste, and that you can train your taste buds to be satisfied with less and less sugar. As you begin to get away from your crutch foods, you can find more healthful ways to deal with your emotions, rather than sugarcoating them, so to speak, with unhealthful foods. Again, the only way to permanently relieve the stress, anger, or sadness in your life is to deal with the source of these emotions. But, until then, healthy indulgences are key.

WHEN YOU NEED SOMETHING TO DO WITH YOUR HANDS

People will often eat just to have something to do while they watch TV. That's why movie concession stands do so well, despite the shameless price gouging. It's not that those stale bins of candy are so great tasting, but once you've hit the third hour of *Lord of the Rings*, you start to get a bit antsy. You're barely paying any attention to what you're putting in your mouth, because your brain is on automatic pilot.

Instead of completely passive, sedentary activities such as TV watching, why not try some other indoor pastimes that engage the mind and hands a lot more, leaving you less vulnerable to mindless indulging?

Play Board Games

It may seem old-fashioned, but playing Boggle, Pictionary, charades, Trivial Pursuit, Scattergories, or any other group game is a great way to spend time with friends. Not only are these games entertaining (Pictionary requires its players to draw clues for their team, and it's hilarious making fun of the pathetic stick figures created by your peers), but you get to know people a lot better when you actually interact with them during a competitive game of Connect Four than you ever would have done sitting next to them in a darkened theater.

Do a Crossword

Dorky as this may sound, doing a crossword is a really great way to stay sharp and increase your vocabulary and knowledge of random factoids. You keep your mind off food and your hands out of the cookie jar—because crosswords are challenging and fun. Trust me, trying to come up with an eight-letter word for "puzzle" will wipe everything else from your mind. (Try "quandary.") You can find crosswords at most major pharmacies and convenience stores, and in many weekend newspapers.

Start Knitting

Knitting is the new yoga for Hollywood stars. Homemade clothing creations are popping up on starlets, and their minute pooches, up and down the coasts. This is one Hollywood pastime you can afford (jetting off to the south of France might be higher on your list, but you have to play with the cards you're dealt). Not only is knitting easy and inexpensive to pick up, it keeps those little hands busy for hours at a time. You can also create beautiful objects and gifts, so that you have something to show for your efforts. You can purchase knitting materials and beginner books at any local craft shop.

Go for a Walk

Going for a walk is a wonderful way to get exercise any time of day—alone, or with your companion of choice. It's a fun way to explore your campus or the surrounding area, so you learn something new and won't even remember that you're exercising *and* avoiding overeating. You can have just as productive and satisfying a conversation while moving your arms and legs as you would yakking and sharing a plate of greasy fries at a snack bar. It may even be a more productive conversation, as walking in the fresh air will clear your head and increase alertness.

Play Games

And I don't mean computer games. Old-fashioned, physical games like hide-and-seek, capture the flag, snowball fights (weather permitting), manhunt (a personal favorite), and other conventional camp games are a blast and a terrific way to meet people in interesting places. They're great for burning off calories, too. Check out the rules online, or make up your own.

The first snow of last year, we got about three inches. It wasn't much, but six of us got together and had a boys-vs.-girls snowball showdown; we were sprinting through the snow, slipping all over, getting sopping wet, and being pelted with what were fast becoming ice balls. By the time we all finally collapsed into a huddle of freezing bodies on the common room floor, we were panting and exhausted—and incredibly happy. We ended up making great memories on a night that could have been spent uneventfully watching yet another movie. These are just a few ways I found to get my hands and body moving so that I wouldn't fall into the trap of mindless overeating. Find ways to enjoy a free minute with friends or pick up a new skill, and pretty soon, you won't even miss your spot on the floor in front of the tube.

SMOKING AND DRINKING: ACTIVITIES THAT KILL

Kids in high school often fantasize about the freedom college offers. The idea of living on your own with a bunch of friends for four years tends to block out any thoughts of a hefty courseload or, even worse, a hefty Freshman 15. Naturally, with so much freedom being foisted upon young-and-impressionables all at once, some tend to go overboard. With all the experimenting that goes on in college (and no, I'm not talking about the potion you whipped up in Chemistry 101), some individuals find themselves adopting habits they were never inclined to before entering college.

Smoking and alcohol abuse (also known as binge drinking if you have more than four drinks in a sitting) are two very common habits that are easy to pick up in college, and that, if you're not careful, can remain with you throughout life. When you're young, you have a generalized sense of immortality. Your young body seems to bounce back from just about anything, short of a nuclear blast. But rest assured, your habits will catch up with you. College students drink an estimated 430 million gallons of alcohol yearly. That's enough to fill an Olympic-size pool for each

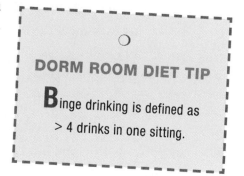

DORM ROOM DIET TIP

Binge drinking is defined as > 4 drinks in one sitting.

college and university in the United States. Unfortunately, as many as 360,000 of the nation's 12 million undergraduates will ultimately die from alcohol-related causes.

Now, my father's a doctor, so I have known all about the dangers of smoking cigarettes since I was a very little girl. My father was always more of a shower than a teller, so when I was an adolescent, he took me into the operating room with him one day when he was doing a heart transplant on a fifty-year-old male who had been a lifelong smoker. This man's insides were disgusting: his lungs were purple-black and, rather than being smooth like a healthy lung, they were lumpy from all the cigarette tar. It was a revolting sight, and the man's suffering as a result of his smoking was even more compelling. Here he was, undergoing open-heart surgery, and his sickness was probably completely preventable. It made me think twice about how important the decisions we make daily can be.

In addition to decaying, mottled insides, smokers can look forward to premature aging, wrinkles, sallow skin, brown teeth, and bad breath—there for all the world to see and smell every day of your life.

Let's face it: being a smoker today is inconvenient, to say the least. In the United States, recent legislation makes it impossible for you to smoke indoors in most places. And being dependent on tobacco can really cramp your style, not to mention your budget. (At nearly $10 a pack, who wants that avoidable expense?) Once you are addicted to the nicotine in cigarettes, it's extremely difficult to quit. If you don't have your nicotine fix you'll feel cranky, have a headache, and basically get a self-induced form of a head cold. People have been able to quit, but there is no easy way and those who do succeed have to endure weeks, if not months, of suffering to get over a self-imposed, debilitating habit. I'm sure you've heard all the smoking cons before, but I'm having a really hard time trying to think of a pro list. It could be because there aren't any pros.

Even with all these drawbacks, 51 percent of college students say they are social smokers, meaning that they smoke with other people to fit in, not because they are addicted. Yet, in 2002 there were 45.8 million people over the age of eighteen in the United States who smoked, meaning some of these social smokers must have picked up a dependency. Some of my friends who are smokers have tried to convince me that they started smoking to help themselves lose weight. My response to this is that smoking kills *and* it makes you ugly. There are plenty of ways to lose weight that don't require sacrificing your health or your looks.

Alcohol abuse is a whole other topic. Lawn parties, frat parties, club parties—you can find a party any night of the week, if you're looking. And the majority of these are not sit-down get-togethers where you share a nice bottle of chardonnay among friends. These are full-blown, drink-beer-till-you-barf parties.

> As many as 1,400 students die each year from alcohol-related causes, including falls and car accidents

Hospitalization (and, in the worst cases, death) from acute alcohol poisoning or alcohol-related accidents is known to occur on college campuses. Research suggests that an astounding 1,400 students die each year from alcohol-related causes, including falls and car accidents.

If the possibilities of severely impaired judgment and even death don't scare you, take the time to think about the extra calories you consume in one of these late-night drinking competitions—about 100 calories in even a light beer. Every once in a while, adding a little alcohol to the mix is fine (unless you're under twenty-one, when drinking is a crime punishable by jail time, license revocation, and/or steep fines). But the excess with which so many young adults drink not only makes them fat but harms their physical appearance in other ways. Excessive drinking puts abusers at risk for premature wrinkling, undereye bags, straggly hair, and a sickly complexion. Drinking also puts them at risk for liver decay, heart failure, and stroke: think about that the next time someone offers to tap you one.

I know it's unrealistic to hope that showering you with statistics about the kind of damage you can do to your own body—the same one you are working hard to feed healthfully—will keep you from experimenting a little with cigarettes and alcohol (after all, nothing is off limits!). But I do hope this information sticks in your mind and gets you through some of the tough decisions you'll undoubtedly face in college.

So we've now dealt with the energy input side of the equation. What about the energy output half? You can only lose weight if you are taking in less energy than you are expending. So now it's time to learn how to work out, even on the tightest of schedules, in the smallest of dorm rooms.

STEP 6

GET MOVING

The Exercise Factor

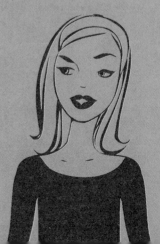

" I have a love-hate relationship with exercise. I positively dread going to the gym: I despise the idea of sweating in public, loathe exercising in cramped spaces, and consider the superfit girl whizzing along on the elliptical next to me my nemesis. But after I get past all the moaning and groaning, and the reluctance to do my full workout, I always leave feeling great. I love the flushed glow I get postworkout, the soreness in my muscles the next day—I've even forgiven that little roadrunner her sin of being in better shape than I am. In fact, she's become my new best friend, because she's just the motivation I need to go back tomorrow, and the next day."

—ANNA, 21

L IKE ANNA, LOTS of people have a love-hate relationship with exercise. Exercising is a commitment, and not an easy one at that. It requires time, energy, dedication, not to mention a thick skin. Sometimes you'll look completely spastic (the elliptical is a hard machine to look coordinated on, let me tell you). Thankfully, exercise gets a lot easier as you become more accustomed to a weekly routine and feel inspired by gradual changes in your shape. But deciding which program (or programs) will work best for you, and then sticking to your plans despite all the distractions on campus, can be a real challenge to most college students. Luckily, the rewards are substantial.

WHY IS EXERCISE SO IMPORTANT?

First of all, exercise helps you to get in or stay in shape. It helps build muscle, increasing your metabolism so you burn off more calories, even when you are resting. An hour of strenuous, aerobic exercise, such as running, speed walking, or dancing, can burn more than 500 calories. A pound of fat is 3,500 calories. Just imagine the havoc you could wreak on your muffin top or midriff with five hours of aerobic exercise per week!

Exercise also enhances your immune system and boosts brain power. By pumping blood to your brain and the rest of your body, exercise increases your alertness and concentration. This means that the forty-five minutes you spend exercising may actually better prepare you for tomorrow's test (by keeping your brain focused and your studying efficient) than if you had spent that time studying or taking a break to refuel with a snack. Exercise is also a great way to improve your mood, because sustained physical activity causes your body to produce endorphins (remember those "happy" chemicals?). That's why you feel vibrant and energetic after you swim, run, or work out.

Then there are the social benefits of exercising. Exercise limits the amount of time you can spend overeating, smoking, drinking alcohol, or doing other potentially health-harming things you'll later regret. The gym is also a great place to meet new people who are also interested in taking care of their bodies. So, you'll be boosting your self-esteem on two levels: you'll like your body even more once you start to get in shape, and your new friends will provide you with a circle of support should you start to fall off the exercise bandwagon.

And there's more. Let's quickly summarize the benefits of exercise:

1. LOOKING BETTER

➤ tones your muscles and increases BMR (see Step 2)

➤ burns off calories to help lose extra pounds or helps you stay at your desirable weight

➤ helps control your appetite

➤ increases blood circulation so your skin gets all the nutrients it needs and maintains a youthful glow from the inside out; also, you sweat out impurities through the pores in your skin, which helps keep your body clear of toxins

2. WORKING BETTER

➤ helps you to be more productive at school and/or work

➤ increases your capacity for physical work

➤ makes you more alert and focused

➤ increases muscle strength

➤ helps your heart and lungs work more efficiently

3. FEELING BETTER

- ➤ gives you more energy

- ➤ improves your self-image

- ➤ increases resistance to fatigue

- ➤ helps counter stress, anxiety, and depression

- ➤ helps you to relax and feel less tense

- ➤ improves your ability to fall asleep quickly and sleep well

- ➤ provides an easy way to socialize with friends or family and an opportunity to meet new friends

With all these obvious benefits, why isn't everyone on campus lifting and sweating every chance they get? We tend to think of exercise as inconvenient, sometimes embarrassing, and even boring. But there is also the fear of failure: we're afraid that we'll commit to a program and won't stick to it or won't feel adequately rewarded for our efforts. This is a completely legitimate concern: sometimes the weight does take a while to come off—especially if you cheat a little, either by eating unhealthy things or skimping on exercise time. In order to keep up the good work, you need to provide yourself with small bonuses: use exercise as a time for introspection, make it fun, and be sure to give yourself little rewards for each milestone you reach.

Let's look at two of the most common reasons students give for not getting the exercise they need.

"Exercising Is Boring"

Running in place for twenty minutes may not sound like your idea of excitement, but there are ways to make it more fun. Listen to a Walkman, or the ubiquitous iPod. If your gym has a television, watch that. Read a magazine, newspaper article, or that novel for English you've been putting off. Many people find that they are most creative when exercising, so use the time to think about problems you're trying to figure out. Solutions might just pop into your head.

Most schools now have clean, well-equipped sports facilities right on campus, which are open to you with the cost of tuition. Use them—you're paying for them anyway. But keep in mind that you don't have to exercise indoors or in a gym. Pick an activity that you like and are good at (for example, soccer, bike riding, shooting hoops) and either play a pickup game, or just practice on your own. If you like competition, maybe you'll want to take a martial arts class. If you're looking for camaraderie, a running league or an intramural team at your college might be right for you. If you just like to be on your own without distraction from others, swimming laps is a really good option. If you want to relax and get centered while you exercise, try a yoga routine. Or, if you want to see the sweat pour, try a kickboxing class; it's like swimming, without the pool. Whatever you choose, remember to keep it interesting *and* challenging. Once your old workout stops getting you out of breath, it's time to up the intensity or try something new for a while so that your body doesn't get too comfortable and stop burning calories effectively.

A great way to encourage yourself to exercise is to set up a system of goals and rewards. "Losing weight" is not specific enough: there are no defined parameters, no breakpoints at which you can stop and pat yourself on the back. "Losing three pounds" is more defined, but you still don't have a time line. "I want to lose three pounds in two weeks" is an achievable goal with finite parameters. Once you've set a good goal, pick out a small reward (just not food!)—maybe a pedicure or a cute skirt to go with your slimmer physique—for when you've achieved it. If you don't achieve your goal by the set time, create a new goal. You don't get the big reward you had planned until you reach your goal, so you still have an incentive. But if you've lost two pounds by the end of week 2, that definitely merits some music downloads or another small treat. Make sure you reward yourself appropriately for work well done, and you'll have no reason to abandon your goals.

"But I Don't Have Time to Exercise!"

I sympathize with this plea, I really do. I know how tough it is to get your schedule planned so that you have time to exercise, shower, and so on, what with classes, extra meetings with professors, and coffee with that guy you met last week at your friend's birthday party. But that's when you thought exercise had to involve a two-hour fight with the machines at the gym. Not only does exercise not have to take two hours; it doesn't even have to be in a gym. Walking to the library to study instead of staying in your dorm or simply going to the bathroom on a different floor from your classroom or dorm room are excellent ways to work more movement (and energy expenditure) into your day. (See the exercise routine at the end of the chapter for other easy in-dorm energy boosters.) Wearing a pedometer (a small, practically weightless device that you clip onto your waistband) enables you to count the number of steps you take per day, so that you can consciously make an effort to raise this number. (Aim for 10,000 a day and watch the pounds drop and the endurance climb.)

The easiest way I know to make time for exercise is to get it over with in the morning. Not only do you rev up your energy for the rest of the day, but you then don't have to think about exercising again until tomorrow. It's already out of the way, taken care of, end of discussion. If you just can't muster the energy to get out of bed an hour early (depending on when your first class is), set aside an hour in the late afternoon when you know nothing is usually going on (the hour before dinner is good) and get to the gym. Keep in mind that a strenuous exercise session too close to your bedtime can interfere with sleep. You'll have to look at your own schedule and see when exercising works for you.

Exercise does not need to take over your life if you don't let it. Resolve to get some physical activity in each day and then do it. No ifs, ands, or buts. After a while, you won't even have to consider whether or not you have to exercise today. It will become automatic, like brushing your teeth. The key thing here is not to make exercise a burden, or it will silently work itself out of your life.

Maybe I'm preaching to the choir. Maybe you already want to start an exercise routine, already know it would be good for you if you did. Don't plan to start getting healthy someday . . . do it now. Yes, right now. Put the book down and jog in place for five minutes. That's right, stop reading! STEP AWAY FROM THE BOOK. (But don't forget to come back when you're done . . . I have a surprise for you.)

So, how was it? If you were too out of shape to jog for five minutes, use that as an added incentive to start a workout routine immediately. If five minutes of jogging was a piece of cake, great! You should feel energized and alert after your brief workout. And, here's the surprise, you've already burned about 50 calories. Just think, ten brief workouts like this a day and you'll have burned 500 calories. A week of these workouts and you'll have burned 3,500 calories—equivalent to a pound of fat. Now that goal doesn't seem all that distant, does it?

CREATING AN EXERCISE PLAN

Just as there isn't one goal for everyone who exercises, there isn't a one-size-fits-all exercise for everybody out there. Some people want to lose weight, so they do primarily cardio workouts—that is, workouts that raise their heart and breathing rates for a sustained period of time. Some exercisers want to tone specific body parts, so they primarily do bodywork (like crunches, pull-ups, push-ups, and other weight-bearing activities). Some want to change the form of their bodies, so they do strength training (weight lifting) that forces their muscles to change shape and build. Some exercise to help them relax and relieve stress, so they might choose a less strenuous form of exercise, such as yoga. But to get the best body possible (we're talking slim, toned, and relaxed—all at the same time), you need to vary your exercise routine so that your body doesn't get used to one type of workout and stop responding to your efforts.

How does this happen? Your body is really smart. If it knows exactly what to expect every time you exercise, it can figure out ways to do the work without having to expend as much energy, or otherwise adjust to the motions you're putting it through. If you do the same routine over and over again, you work the same muscle groups continuously. At first they'll respond to the new workout by building strength, endurance, and tone. But, eventually, your muscles will plateau at the level of strength, endurance, and tone that a particular level of workout can elicit. That's why it's important to vary the muscle groups you are working, as well as the level at which they are being worked.

This also goes for fat-burning exercises, such as running and using the elliptical machine. If you run two miles every day, you'll see dramatic results at first, but eventually your body will get accustomed to this training and you won't have to work as hard to complete the run. This is when you either have to run farther, change your course (add some hills), or alter your pace (either run faster, steadily, or add some sprints to your jog) to make sure you are still working out effectively. There will never be a point at which you don't burn calories from exercising, but you want to make sure that you are burning as many as possible.

To get a complete body workout, you need to vary not only the *intensity*, but also the *type* of workout. Exchange one day of cardio for a day of strength training or a day of relaxing and lengthening activity, such as yoga. This will not only keep your body guessing, so it takes longer for it to figure out how to economize during the workout, but it also gives you a chance to have some days on which the exercise is light-to-none. We'll get more into specific exercise routines later on in this chapter. But, right now, I want to walk through a basic overall exercise plan with you. We'll work up to thirty minutes to an hour of cardio three days a week, with one hour of strength training one day and one hour of lengthening (such as yoga or Pilates) on another. This leaves you with two days a week when you don't have to exercise at all, if you don't want.

> **DORM ROOM DIET TIP**
>
> Falling off the exercise wagon (say, when your life is insane around finals time) does not mean your exercise routine is as good as dead. Just pick up where you left off as soon as you can.

Your Basic Cardio

Everyone's heard the term "cardio." That's the word your lacrosse coach uses before she explains that you'll be doing a six-mile run followed by a set of sprints. Cardio, which is short for cardiovascular, workouts are usually the ones that burn the most fat, because a cardio workout is one that gets your heart and breathing rates up and keeps them up. Your little jog a few minutes ago was a form of cardio exercise, though it only sped up your heart rate for five minutes. When doing a cardio workout, there is a certain heart rate you want to reach and sustain, so that your body burns fat the most efficiently. This is called your target heart rate (THR). You want to reach a heart rate (the number of heartbeats per minute) within your target heart rate *range* and hold that level for at least half an hour.

CALCULATING YOUR
TARGET HEART RATE RANGE

To determine your target heart rate, subtract your age from 220, then take this number and multiply by 0.6. This is your low limit. Then take the original 220 minus your age number and multiply by 0.85. This is your high limit. At the most intense part of your workout, your heart rate should fall somewhere between these numbers, but never above. When your heart rate exceeds this ideal range, your body switches from aerobic (your body is using oxygen to fuel metabolism to get energy) to anaerobic (your body is using other chemical processes that do not require oxygen to fuel cells—i.e., muscle contractions) exercising, meaning that the cells in your body have switched the source of their energy and will now fatigue faster because anaerobic activity produces waste molecules that impair activity and may make you unable to burn fat as quickly. So, if your heart rate rises above the high limit, slow down.

To figure out what your heart rate is at any given time, place your pointer and middle fingers on your opposite wrist or on your neck, an inch below your ear, so that you can feel your heartbeat. Count the number of beats in fifteen seconds and multiply that number by 4.

When doing a cardio workout, you want to reach your target heart rate and keep it steady. If you're not on a machine that allows you to measure your heart rate, go at a pace that makes you breathe hard, but doesn't leave you so short of breath that you have to stop exercising to catch your breath. Now keep it up for at least half an hour. No, this doesn't mean you'll have to start off with a thirty-minute run right at the beginning of your program. Lifting weights and exercising large muscle groups in quick succession is also considered cardio exercise. Martial arts and kickboxing are also great cardio workouts. So, you could do fifteen minutes on a treadmill or elliptical machine, then get off and immediately go into a weight lifting routine, during which you take thirty seconds to rest between sets of repetitions and a minute break in between each different exercise until you've completed your half-hour.

Go to the gym, talk to a trainer, and take a look around at all the wonderful toys available for your use. Pick something you like and feel challenged by, so you can build it into your weekly routine.

Training Specific Muscle Groups

If you're reading this book primarily to lose weight, not to bulk up your muscles, you may think you only have to do a cardio workout. Doing cardio is an excellent way to get that stubborn scale to start showing the numbers you want. But those shrinking numbers won't be very satisfying if your body isn't becoming more shapely and firm. This is why weight training specific muscle groups is so important to obtaining optimal results.

By training specific muscle groups at varying levels of intensity (to prevent the plateaus we talked about earlier), you can actually get your muscles to take on new shapes and forms. Guys generally go for the bigger is better ideal, whereas women tend to want firm, toned, lean muscles. In either case, you'll need to strength train—meaning you need to have moderate resistance—if you want to change the shape of your body. Training with resistance means that you are applying some added weight (add more weight to build larger muscles) to your muscles so that they have to strain to lift that weight. Essentially, when you weight lift you are creating tiny tears in your muscle tissues. Those tears heal (provided you get enough protein in your diet, drink plenty of water, and sleep) and make your muscles stronger and firmer. If you do lots of repetitions with low resistance, you'll get firm, lean, toned muscles, because you are only tearing them a little bit, whereas, if you do a moderate number of repetitions with a very heavy resistance, you'll get larger muscles.

A good way to fit muscle training into your workout schedule is to alternate days of hard cardio with hard muscle training. Hard muscle training does not mean using a lot of resistance. It means using an appropriate weight for your muscle-building goals, but then doing lots of repetitions and taking limited, short breaks. In other words, you should be sweating by the end of this workout as though you'd spent an equal amount of time doing a low-intensity cardio workout. Say on Monday you do an hour on the elliptical and an abdominal routine, then on Tuesday skip your cardio and fill the time doing three muscle training rotations using twelve different machines (use each machine once, then repeat the cycle two more times). You can choose to have all twelve machines focus on a particular muscle group, like arms. Or you can work any combination of body parts.

Weight lifting machines work large muscle groups, so focus on the areas that you want to get longer, leaner, slimmer, or firmer. Each machine will probably have a detailed description of how it is used and what muscle groups it defines, so be sure to use these guides when you are first learning how to use the different machines. Using free weights is also a great way to tone specific body areas. Because free weights train small muscle groups, you should start with the bigger muscle groups (using machines) so that you don't get burned out in the beginning by overworking the little guys.

On Wednesday, go back to your cardio. You can adjust this routine if you feel yourself getting too sore from your iron-pumping sessions. Do a day of light cardio instead of a weight training session to give yourself a break. Also, on a light exercise day or any time, you can pick up a can of soup or that giant calculus book and do a few sets of lifts to tone your muscles without leaving the comfort of your dorm room. Later in this chapter, I will explain a variety of different workout schedules and plans, so you can choose which configuration works best for you.

Lengthening and Strengthening Workouts

Yoga and Pilates are exercises that have been absorbed into our culture, but may still have an air of mystique about them. Both are great workouts that allow you to build and tone long, lean muscle. Yoga does this by making you lift your own body weight in a variety of positions, so your own weight provides the resistance for strength training. It has its roots in ancient Indian practices of meditation, so the focus of yoga is to achieve equanimity, or evenness of mind. (Basically, you're supposed to learn how to be comfortable with being uncomfortable—some of the positions into which yogis can contort their bodies are not exactly easy, but the idea is to have your mental calm overcome this state of physical strain.) Yoga strengthens all parts of your body. Pilates, on the other hand, is a core workout, which means that it focuses on strengthening and tightening the muscles in your torso (your "core") to improve posture and lengthen your spine.

It used to be that these sorts of workout routines only appealed to the adventurous ex-hippies among us. But now that mainstream Western culture, and Hollywood, has made yoga so trendy and ubiquitous, you can get involved without feeling as if you're the only person under fifty in the room. With cardio exercise you move your muscles quickly, an action that shortens and tightens your muscles (giving you that great sore feeling after a hard workout); with traditional yoga you move your muscles slowly, lengthening and loosening them. Toning and building muscle mass with cardio exercise is healthy because muscles burn more calories than fat, thereby increasing your metabolism. But with all the tension and stress in your life as a college student, you need to take time to quiet down your body and give it a chance to rejuvenate. During lengthening and stretching workouts, instead of rushing to your muscles as it does in cardio exercising, your blood is free to do repair work throughout the body.

There are different types of yoga workouts available, some of which feel more like cardio than relaxation. Power yoga and yoga done in rooms at extremely high temperatures, called Bikram yoga, still move your muscles slowly, but involve much more strenuous poses that really build muscle rather than relaxing it. So you can use yoga to build, tone, or to relax and rejuvenate muscle groups, depending on your needs.

Yoga studios and classes are a great way to get started on yoga, since you will want a professional instructor to show you if you are doing the various *asanas*, or poses, correctly. Starting out on your own can be risky, since you will be doing some poses that, if done incorrectly, could potentially harm your neck, back, and shoulders. In yoga you are trying to learn how to be comfortable with being uncomfortable, but this most definitely does not include being uncomfortable while you snap your neck. So try a few classes and then feel free to take off on your own. There are plenty of books and DVDs that can help you deepen your practice, once you've got the basics down. The great thing about these workouts is they are relaxed enough that you can do them even in the confined space of your dorm.

Pilates is a slightly different breed of lengthening exercise. Since the practice was actually derived from a routine for ballerinas—and we all know how firm-but-feminine those ladies are—the kind of muscle you'll be building won't bulk you up. The Pilates workout has several variations. The traditional version, called mat Pilates, feels like light stretching combined with an abdominal routine, but the more intense version (which involves specifically designed machines in a Pilates studio, called a tower) will leave you dripping more sweat than if you had spent the last hour running in 100-degree weather. Now there are some videos you use to learn the basic Pilates principles. But, unless you are much luckier than I am, your dorm room probably isn't big enough to incorporate all the equipment you need to have a really strenuous Pilates workout, so see if you can find a studio or a class to join near your college. Otherwise, check out amazon.com or barnesandnoble.com for some in-home routines.

Stretching

It's crucial that you stretch after a workout. Stretching your muscles will help them get rid of lactic acid, a by-product of the processes that go on in your body to give you energy during a hard workout. A concentration of lactic acid can lead to muscle cramps. In any case, you want to be sure to stretch and drink plenty of water to flush this toxin out of your body and aid your muscles in the healing process. Many trainers believe that you should stretch both before *and* after your workout so that you have blood pumping through your muscles before you attempt any strenuous activity.

Stretching is *not* a quick plunge to touch the floor with your fingers and then back up. Nor is it a bouncing, bent-over version of the same thing. To really stretch, you need to hold three, thirty-second stretches in each form. Don't skip stretching because you don't mind (or maybe even like) feeling sore after a hard workout. Have no fear; you'll be able to feel the workout even after stretching (assuming you worked out hard enough). What you won't get if you don't stretch is nice, long, lean muscles. Not stretching can cause muscles to stay tight, adding bulk rather than length.

WORKOUT

Many girls underestimate the importance of weight lifting in their weekly workout schedules. Sure, most girls don't want to look like bodybuilders, but the toning, tightening, and strengthening effects of light strength training are results no girl wants to pass up. So, what happens when you can't make it to the gym but still want to up the blood flow to the various core muscle groups: chest and triceps, legs, back, biceps, and abdominals (abs)? Well, with the help of Joel Harper, a celebrity fitness trainer and yoga instructor in New York City, I've put together five, fifteen-minute routines— each focused on one of the core muscle groups—that you can do in the comfort of your own dorm room. Within each group is a series of strength exercises that allow you to use your own body weight as resistance: this way you build tone rather than mass (think supermodel instead of the Incredible Hulk). I've also included intermittent stretches in each set. Stretching is a really crucial part of any workout routine because it helps get and keep the muscles warm so that you get better results. Also, stretching elongates the muscle you are building, so that you don't bulk up.

Getting Started

Before you start your strength training routine, find yourself a flight of stairs. A few stair climber moves will give your muscles a quick boost of blood and heat to prepare them for your workout. Start on a landing. Step up two steps with your right foot and bring your left foot up to meet it. Step back down to the landing with your left foot first and bring your right foot down to meet it. Repeat this activity, this time with your left foot stepping up first. Do this 60 times to really get the blood flowing before you embark on any serious stretching or muscle exercising.

Next, roll your shoulders 10 times forward, 10 times backward, and then make 20 full circles with your arms out to the side, back 10 times and forward 10 times. With your feet firmly on the floor, hold your arms straight out to the side and swing your upper body in a circle by bending to the front, side, and back to rotate your hips 10 times in each direction.

For every exercise that follows, proper breathing is essential. Do not hold your breath; inhale on the lift and exhale on the release. Be aware of tightening in other parts of your body—the most common areas are the face and shoulders. Try to remain relaxed and isolate the muscle being worked.

Let's get started with your five basic, in-dorm workout routines.

Chest and Triceps

UPPER PUSH-UP Lie down on your stomach and put your hands palms down and shoulder-width apart on the floor. Push up so that your body is flat like a board, your arms are extended, and your toes are on the floor. Hold this position for 30 seconds, remembering not to let your butt push up into the air. Keep your stomach pulled in to support your lower back.

Lie on your stomach and rest for 30 seconds.

LOWER PUSH-UP While still lying on your stomach, place your palms on the floor underneath each of your armpits. Push your body up to the upper push-up position, then lower your body so that your chest is about 6 inches off the floor and your back is straight (make sure your butt is not sticking up in the air!). Hold this position for 30 seconds. Repeat 4 times.

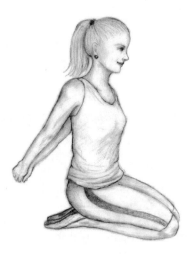

CHEST STRETCH Sit on your heels, interweave your fingers behind your back, and lift your chest up 10 times by inhaling.

GIRL PUSH-UPS With your knees on the floor and your ankles lifted and crossed, do 10 push-ups. Repeat 2 times.

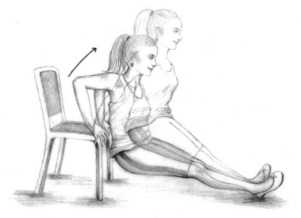

CHAIR DIPS Find a stationary chair and squat in front of it. Put your palms on the seat of the chair behind you and grip it so that you're clasping the front of the chair. While holding yourself up, walk your feet out in front of you until your legs are straight and you are resting on your palms and heels. Now lift your body up with your arms and then lower it 10 times. Hold the final lower dip for 30 seconds.

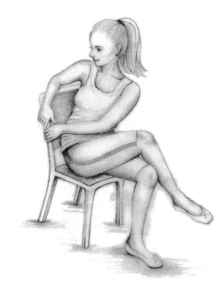

BACK STRETCH Sit in a chair and cross your right leg over your left. Twist your torso and try to place both your right and left hands on the back of the chair. If this is too much of a stretch, put your left hand on the right corner of the chair and clasp the back of the chair with your right hand only. Hold the stretch for 30 seconds. Repeat on the other side.

TRICEPS STRETCH Lift your right arm over your head, bending at the elbow, as if to scratch the middle of your back. Press your right elbow down with your left palm until you feel a moderate stretch.

CHAIR DIPS Do 10 more chair dips, holding the final lower dip for 30 seconds.

TRICEPS STRETCH Reach across your chest with your right arm and bend your left arm at the elbow and use it to pull your right arm tight into your body.

DOWN DOG INCLINE CHEST PUSH-UPS (This move is taken from a basic yoga routine.) Start off by standing with your feet flat on the floor and bend over to touch the floor. Put your palms flat on the floor, bending at the knees if you need to. Then walk your feet out behind you until you are in a pyramid position, with your palms on the floor and your feet as close to flat on the floor as possible. The trick to this pose is to push back into your heels so that you feel a stretch (not an ouch!) in the back of your thighs (hamstrings); you will simultaneously be working the muscles in your upper arms and shoulders. Depending on how flexible you are, you might need to come up onto your toes to relieve the stretch in your hamstrings. Slowly bring your body parallel to the floor by walking your feet backward. Bend your arms, keeping your elbows close to your sides, and lower your body to about an inch off the floor. Hold for 5 seconds. Then go back to the down dog (pyramid) position by walking your feet forward again. Repeat this 10 times.

Legs

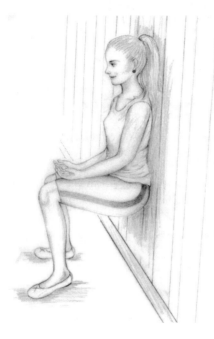

HUMAN CHAIR Press your back against a wall with your legs bent at a 90-degree angle, as if you were sitting in a chair. Hold this position for 1 minute. Make sure your knees stay directly above your ankles.

TOE TOUCH Stand with your feet flat on the floor and bend at the waist, keeping your legs and back as straight as possible; try to touch your toes. If you need a better stretch, try laying your hands flat on the floor, palms facing down. Breathe through your lower back. Scan your body; wherever you feel tension, release. Use the weight of your head and shoulders to elongate your spine.

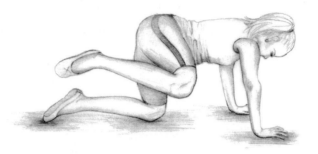

SIDE LEG LIFT Position yourself with all fours on the floor, knees shoulder-width apart and palms facing down. Keeping your knee bent, lift your right leg out to the side until it is nearly level with your back and then lower it to the starting position. Repeat 50 times, and do another 50 lifts with your left leg. If this is hard or uncomfortable on your wrists, lower down to your elbows. In either position keep your stomach pulled in, supporting your lower back. Focus on isolating your butt muscle.

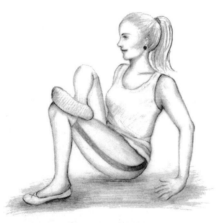

BUTT STRETCH Sit down and bring your feet as close to your butt as possible, slightly less than shoulder-width apart. Put your hands, palms down and fingers facing forward, a couple of inches behind you and push your bottom a few inches up off the floor. Cross your right leg over your left knee so that your right ankle rests just above your left kneecap. Lower your butt toward the floor to increase the stretch. Lightly press your lower back up toward the calf of the leg that is crossed. Think elongating your spine instead of compacting it down. Switch sides. Breathing and relaxing are key.

BACK KICK Flip over and get back on your hands and knees. Keeping your knees bent, use your right butt cheek and pull the sole of your right foot up toward the ceiling, making a 45-degree angle. Repeat 50 times. Don't arch your back; keep your stomach in to support your lower back. Complete another 50 kicks with your left leg.

STRAIGHT LEG STRETCH Sit on the floor, straighten your legs in front of you, ankles touching. Interlace your thumbs and lean forward so that you are as close to gripping your feet as possible. Grip them if you can. Hold this position for 20 seconds. Remember that this stretch needs to be continuous, no bouncing or fidgeting; if touching your toes is too uncomfortable, just go as far as you can.

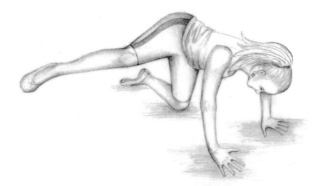

SIDE KNEE KICK Get back in your side lift position. This time, instead of just lifting your leg up and lowering it back to the starting position, at the top of your lift you are going to extend your leg out to the side of your body while tensing your leg muscles. Kick 25 times and switch legs. Your knee stays in the same position during the kicks. Your lower leg is the only thing that moves.

HALF BUTTERFLY TOE TOUCH While sitting, bend your right knee and pull your heel into your body while extending your left leg, pointing your toes toward the ceiling. Lean forward and touch your toes with your left hand; use the other hand to elongate your spine and keep your body upright. Hold for 30 seconds. Switch sides.

INNER LEG LIFT Lie on your right side. Bend your left leg over your right leg, place your left foot flat on the floor, and hold your ankle with your left hand; support your upper body by coming up onto your right elbow. Keeping your foot perpendicular to your leg (*not* pointing), lift your right leg 50 times. Switch sides and do another 50 lifts.

LEG LIFT Sit with your legs in front of you. Bend your left leg up and interweave your fingers on the opposite side of that knee—this is to help you sit up straight. Take the right leg with foot flexed and pointed straight up and lift it 6 inches off the floor. Keep it straight. Tap the floor and come back up. Repeat 50 times and switch sides.

BUTTERFLY Just as you did in kindergarten, sit down and bring the flats of your feet against each other. Use your hands to pull your heels as close into your body as possible, while keeping your knees close to the floor.

Hold for 30 seconds—elongate your spine. Pretend there is a string on top of your head, pulling your head up as your lower back moves toward your heels.

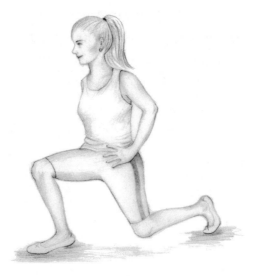

LUNGES Stand upright with your hands on your hips. Keep your back erect and shoulders pressed down (elongate your neck). Step 2 feet in front of you with your right foot and bend both knees so that your left knee comes to an inch above the floor. Come back to standing position by pushing up with your thighs and bringing your right foot back to the starting position (next to your left foot). Alternate between stepping with your right and left leg until you have completed a total of 50 lunges. It is very important to keep your forward knee directly over the ankle.

QUAD PULL Standing upright, bend your right leg and grasp your ankle behind your back with both hands. This also helps improve your balance. Hold the stretch for 30 seconds. Switch sides.

CALF LIFT Stand upright and, with toes pointing forward, lift up onto your toes. Come back to starting position. Repeat 25 times. Come back to the starting position and point your toes in toward each other at about a 45-degree angle. Repeat the calf lift. Come back to the starting position. Face your toes out at about a 45-degree angle, heels touching, and repeat. Come back to the starting position. With your toes facing forward, lift your heels up as high as you can and hold for 30 seconds.

CALF STRETCH While standing up, climb your toes up a wall, so that your foot is as close to flat against the wall as is comfortable. Lean into the wall with your body to increase the stretch in your calf. Repeat with the other leg.

Back

LEG AND OPPOSITE ARM LIFT Kneel on all fours. Extend one leg and the opposite arm in opposite directions and hold for 1 minute. Switch sides.

BACK STRETCH Lie on your back, tuck your knees into your chest, and clasp your arms around your legs by holding on to your elbows. Pull your knees into your chest. Keep your ankles uncrossed. Press your tailbone into the carpet, which will pull your elbows higher and give you a shoulder stretch as well. Elongate your spine. Hold for 30 seconds.

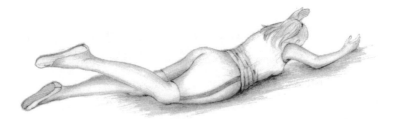

HYPEREXTENSIONS ("THE TODDLER") Lie down on your stomach with your arms stretched out in front of you. Arch your back and lift one leg and the opposite arm. Alternate 25 times. Rest for 10 seconds. Repeat twice. For a more advanced version, swim with both arms and legs off the floor while you switch back and forth.

LEG PULLS Lie on your stomach, bend your knees, and grasp both ankles with your hands. Use your leg strength and slowly lift your shoulders off the floor by pushing your legs back. Hold for 30 seconds.

THE TWIST On all fours, do the same motion as the leg and opposite arm lift. But this time, after extending the opposite leg and arm in opposite directions, bring them back into your body so that the elbow and kneecap gently tap and then extend again. Return to starting position and repeat 25 times. Switch sides.

BACK STRETCH Lie on your back. Grab one knee with the opposite arm and bring it across your body while keeping your chest open by extending the other arm in the opposite direction. Breathe and sink down toward the mat. Switch sides.

Shoulders and Biceps

TENNIS BALL TWISTS Stand up tall and stretch your arms out in front of you, making sure to keep your shoulders from rising up; keep your neck long and shoulders down throughout all these shoulder exercises. Pull your stomach in and slightly bend your knees. Curl your tailbone in and tighten your butt. Clench your hands as though each was gripping a tennis ball (or actually grab two, if you have them handy). While tensing your hands, twist them outward and then inward. Continue for 1 minute.

PALMS-UP CROSS In the same position, unclench your hands and face your palms up. Cross your hands back and forth over and under each other at a moderate pace for 1 minute.

PALMS-DOWN CROSS In the same position, face your palms down, and repeat the previous exercise for 1 minute.

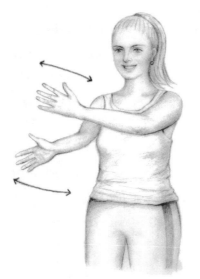

PALMS-IN CROSS In the same position, turn your palms toward each other and cross them back and forth over and under each other for 1 minute. When you start to burn, take deep breaths, breathing into the burn.

RELEASE AND ROLL SHOULDERS Drop your hands to your sides and rotate your shoulders in small circles, 10 times backward and then 10 times forward.

ELBOWS TOGETHER Standing upright with your shoulders down, bend your arms at the elbows and bring your two elbows together so that your palms and forearms are touching and your fingers are pointing to the ceiling. Maintaining this position, lift your arms 1 inch up and 1 inch down for 2 minutes.

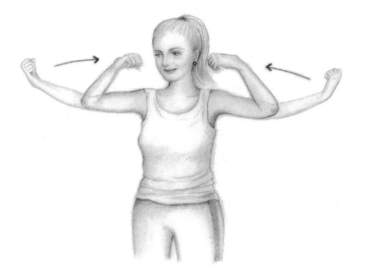

BICEPS CURLS Pretend you are holding dumbbells and stand with your arms out to either side of your body and bent at the elbow, so your elbows are even with your shoulders. While tensing your arm muscles, extend your arms and then bring them back to the upright position 60 times.

BUTT LIFT Sit down, extend your legs in front of you, and place your palms facedown at your sides. Lift your body up and hold for 1 minute. Rest for 15 seconds, and repeat twice.

ARM BALANCE Sit cross-legged, place your palms facedown at your sides, and lift your body off the floor for 10 seconds. Rest 10 seconds, and repeat

3 times. Use your core strength. If it's too hard to hold your entire body off the floor, just hold your butt off.

SHOULDER STRETCH Sit with your legs extended in front of you. Grasp your right leg with your left arm and look over your right shoulder. Hold for 30 seconds and switch sides.

Abdominals

When you're doing abdominal exercises, it's especially important to remember that you never want to use your neck to do the work your core should be doing. If your neck feels strained, cradle your head in your hands like an egg and shift the stress back to your abs. Also, to make sure that you don't end up with compact, crunched abs, stretch after every ab workout. Lie on your stomach, put your hands under your chest and push up to really stretch out all the abdominal muscles. Hold this stretch for 30 seconds, come back to a lying-down position for a 15-second rest, and repeat 3 times.

To work the four different main muscle groups in your abdominal region, I've broken this section into four parts. Each portion focuses on a particular muscle group, so mix and match!

Lower Abs

KNEES BENT LIFT Lying on your back with your arms folded across your chest, knees bent, and feet flat on the floor, use your abs to lift your knees to your chest 30 times.

LEGS STRAIGHT UP Lie on your back with your legs straight up in the air, with your feet flexed so that they are parallel to your body. Interlock your thumbs and reach up to touch your toes 30 times.

BUTT LIFT In the same position as the last exercise, lift your butt 1 inch off the floor. Lift your heels straight up toward the ceiling 30 times. Then combine, lifting your upper body and tailbone simultaneously. Aim to get your tailbone about an inch off the floor with each lift. Repeat 30 times.

ONE LEG UP, ONE LEG DOWN Lie flat on your back with your body stretched stiff like a board and arms crossed over your chest. Keep one leg elongated on the floor and raise the other one so that it is perpendicular to the floor (stretched straight up into the air). Bring the leg that is up in the air back down to the floor and lift the other leg up into the air simultaneously. Alternate 20 times. Really focus on pressing your abs into your lower back and your lower back into the floor.

Obliques

SCISSOR KICKS Lie on your back and lift your outstretched legs between 6 inches and 1 foot off the floor. Extend your toes and cross your legs back and forth across each other 20 times. Then hold your extended legs 1 inch off the floor for 15 seconds. Repeat these exercises 2 times in a row.

CIRCLES Lie on your back with your knees bent and feet on the floor; interweave your hands behind your head. Make circles, by keeping your lower back flat and circling your upper body up to the right and crossing over to the left and circling back down to the mat 20 times. Look up toward the ceiling the entire time. Next set: start to the left and then right 20 times. Do 2 sets of each.

SIDE CRUNCHES Lie on your back with your fingers interlaced behind your head (make sure you don't use them to lift your upper body, only to support your neck). You can also cross your arms on your chest. Bend your knees and bring your legs to one side of your body by twisting your torso. So if you are twisting to the left, your left leg should be resting on the floor. You want your knee to be bent at a 90-degree angle, and your upper body and calves to be as close to parallel as possible (try to keep your back as comfortably close to the floor as you can while you are twisted). Use your abs to bring your upper body up in a crunch and back to the floor 30 times. Switch sides and repeat. Take a 30-second break and repeat both sides twice.

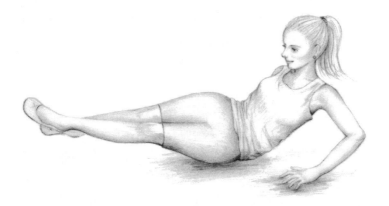

CROSSED LEG LIFT Turn to your side and lift your torso up with your arms while you extend your legs above the floor. Scissor your legs in the air at an angle 20 times. Switch sides and repeat.

Upper Abdominals

ONE-LEG-UP REACH FOR TOE Lie on your back and make a " mountain" with one leg by bending the knee and keeping your foot flat on the floor. Bring your other leg straight up into the air, perpendicular to your chest, and point your toes. Link your thumbs and straighten your arms in front of your body (again, perpendicular to your chest). Lift your upper body as high as you can off the floor (try to touch your foot with your fingertips). Return to a resting position and repeat 20 times. Then repeat on the other side.

45-DEGREE-ANGLE LIFT TOWARD TOE Bend one knee and rest the opposite ankle on this knee. Place your hands behind your head and lift the opposite elbow to the opposite knee. Repeat 20 times. Then repeat on the other side.

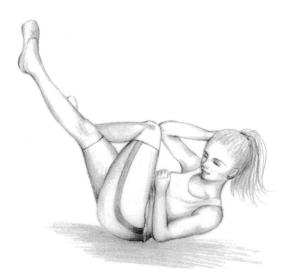

CROSS LEG SHOULDER TWIST Lie on your back with one leg extended up toward the ceiling and the other leg bent and crossed over it. Rest one arm comfortably across your chest or stomach and lightly clasp the back of your neck with the hand of the other arm. Lift your bent elbow to the opposite knee 20 times. Then repeat on the other side.

CROSSED LEG LIFT Turn on your side and lift your torso up with your arms while you extend your legs out above the floor. Lift the leg that is closest to the floor in small, upward kicks, toward the ceiling, in front of the other leg. Repeat 20 times. Then repeat on the other side.

CROSSED ARMS BEHIND HEAD Lying on your back with your feet flat and knees up, cross your arms behind your head making an X, by putting your opposite palm to the opposite shoulder. Rest your head in this X. Your neck should be totally relaxed. Use your abs to lift your upper body off the floor, looking up, and crunch your abs and lower 3 times. Do this twice.

Midsection

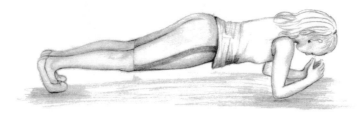

PLANK HOLD Lie on your stomach and raise your straightened body off the floor onto your toes and forearms. Pull your stomach in. Use your oblique muscles to pull your belly button in to support your lower back. Hold for 1 minute.

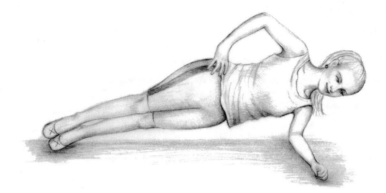

SIDE PLANK In the plank position, open your body up by turning away from the floor so that you face the wall. This requires placing your weight onto one forearm, which may prove too difficult for some of you. If this is the case, just do the regular plank again. Hold for 1 minute.

REGULAR CRUNCHES Lie on your back and make "mountains" with your legs by bending the knees and keeping your feet flat on the floor (your heels should be about a foot from your butt). Interlace your fingers and gently clasp the back of your neck. Use your abs to lift your upper body halfway up to your knees and then back down to the floor and back up to the halfway position (no rests between repetitions). Repeat 40 times, and hold the last crunch in the uppermost position for 1 minute.

KNEE LIFTS Stand up and bend your arms so that your clenched fists or opened palms come in toward your face. Keep your elbows in line with your shoulders. Lift your left knee to meet your left elbow (make sure not to bend your back to make this easier!). Bring your left foot back to the floor and lift your right knee to meet your right elbow. Alternate lifting a knee to its respective elbow 20 times on each side. Repeat twice.

These moves will help you get started with your new workout routine. If you're looking for a more individualized workout without the high cost of a personal trainer, you can go to the Internet and customize your own workout DVD. With www.push.tv/dormroomdiet, for example, you can create a new exercise DVD every month and have it mailed to you.

Whatever you choose, just get moving!

STEP 7

GET YOUR VITAMINS

*Everything You
Need to Know
About Supplements*

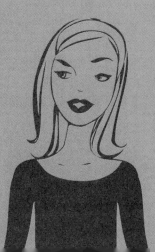

"I grew up taking vitamin and mineral supplements. Once I had teeth, I got chewable tablets with special kid vitamins. When I got older, I started swallowing capsules. It never fazed me to take several pills at one time: just throw 'em in the back of your mouth, take a swig of juice or water, and swallow. Easy. But I'll never forget the day one of my friends slept over and saw the number of vitamins I took each morning and asked, quite sincerely, 'Are you dying?' Naturally, I choked on all the vitamins I'd just tossed into my mouth because I started laughing. And then it dawned on me: some families don't know how important vitamins and minerals can be, even for us healthy folks."

—KARLA, 18

IN CASE YOU didn't grow up on vitamins, or even if you did and are looking for an explanation of why everyone needs a little supplementation now and then, this chapter will provide the answer.

WHAT ARE SUPPLEMENTS?

Vitamins and minerals are tiny chemical compounds your body uses to keep all parts of you healthy. As a product of functioning efficiently, your body produces free radicals, or *oxidants* (products of oxygen molecules), and *antioxidants*, compounds that protect our cell membranes from the harmful effects of oxidative stress (the "rusting" effect oxidants have on our cells). If we didn't have these antioxidants, the free radicals would begin to damage our cells. One result would be premature aging in the form of wrinkles, discolorations, and age spots (which is why you see all these antioxidant face creams around). These same processes are affecting the organs inside your body. If the balance of oxidants and antioxidants in your body is thrown off, you should supplement with additional antioxidants. Obtaining vitamins and minerals from supplements is one way to rebalance the ratio of oxidants to antioxidants, and protect each cell in your body against sickness and infection.

Vitamins and minerals are naturally occurring compounds found in the food we eat. Theoretically, an otherwise healthy person could get all her necessary vitamins and minerals by eating nutrient-dense foods, prepared the right way, eaten in the correct proportions and frequencies. But, in reality, few people do this, especially on a student's schedule and budget. The foods lining convenience store shelves are designed to have the longest shelf life and still look appetizing, not to enhance the nutritional content.

Vitamins and mineral supplements make up for the nutrients you *don't* get from the food you eat; they act as a little insurance policy to make sure you don't fall short. This is especially important for you, the college student, since you need your body to be in top condition to keep up with your course workload, and defend against stress, lack of sleep, and that cougher behind you in Economics. Even though you now know all the foods you *should* be eating daily to get plenty of nutrients, it never hurts to have a backup plan. Certain supplements boost your energy. Others help your immune system to combat a persistent cold. Still others keep your skin smooth, soft, and radiant. You don't want to be caught running low on any of these nutrients.

Be warned, however, that vitamins cannot take the place of food. Just because you take a multivitamin, or five, daily, does not mean you can shovel foods devoid of nutrition into your body and expect to stay healthy. Supplements are called that because they fill in for deficiencies in your day-to-day diet. They are in no way meant to replace a healthy eating regimen.

WHY SHOULD I TAKE SUPPLEMENTS?

There are several reasons why you should be taking supplements. First and most important, they help you acquire and maintain optimal health. Vitamins and minerals keep your bones sturdy, your muscles strong, your hair growing and shiny, and your brain functioning at top speed—all the basic attributes of a healthy human being. They also shield us against illness, and slow down the aging process. Supplements can also be used like medicines to treat and reverse various health problems (without the evil side effects written in fine print on the bottom of your bottle of antacid). Taking vitamins and minerals can prevent nutritional deficiency diseases. These can range in seriousness from skin irritation and bumps due to a lack of essential fatty acids, osteoporosis from mineral deficiency, or even iron-deficiency anemia, a blood condition that is particularly dangerous for menstruating women. During your period, especially if you have a heavy flow, you are losing a variety of fluids, including iron-dense blood. If your diet doesn't include adequate amounts of iron, losing a significant amount each month could lead to iron-deficiency anemia. Anemia means that your blood doesn't have enough red blood cells to transport oxygen adequately. This inadequacy could lead you to feel lethargic and tired constantly.

There are certain supplements that everyone should be taking to maintain basic health. Our bodies don't have the ability to make all the nutrients essential to daily function, so we need to get these crucial nutrients from outside sources. Problem is, with all the processing, microwaving, freezing-and-reheating, freeze-drying, and other crazy things we do to so-called food these days, we aren't getting nearly enough whole foods into our systems. For instance, the flour used to bake white bread is ground from grain that has been stripped of the wheat germ as well as the fibrous shell, thereby depleting its natural fiber and some nutrient content. And every time you perform a cooking process—such as pulling meat apart, grinding it up, squashing it back together in the shape of a kidney, and deep-frying it, as we do with chicken nuggets—you diminish the nutritional value of the food.

The standard American diet—SAD—cries out for supplementation. In the 1930s, a dentist named Weston Price traveled the world documenting the effects of the modern Western diet (excessive protein, lots of processed foods, and too few raw items) on tooth formation and health. He found an increase in tooth decay and crowding (the reason so many American kids wear braces in junior high) in the children of parents who adopted a Western diet. Dr. Price also noticed that these individuals had higher rates of cancer, arthritis, high blood pressure, and tuberculosis—none of which had been present with the non-Western diet previously observed, one that had served people well for millennia. Unfortunately, our diets in this country have strayed even further away from raw, unprocessed items in the decades since Dr. Price's study.

And diet isn't the only factor adversely affecting our health. The harsh environment to which we are exposed damages our bodies in ways you might not be able to see just yet, but that may affect you years from now. Exposure to pollution can actually change the makeup of your DNA. The smallest DNA mutation could be the source of cancers or other diseases later in life. Vitamins interact with each other and also with your own cells through a variety of chemical processes to bolster your body's defenses against free radicals, pollution, and other damaging environmental factors so that you body can function optimally.

Vitamins and natural therapies can also be used to treat a variety of everyday sicknesses. For instance, regular supplementation can boost your immune system, keeping you safe from the common cold and flu. There are supplement solutions for everything from PMS cramps to muscle soreness and from drowsiness to sleeplessness. I'll share some ideas on how to treat some of these common ailments later on in this chapter. But first, let's talk about the human immune system, the primary beneficiary of supplementation.

> **DORM ROOM DIET TIP**
>
> The 1994 Dietary Supplement Health and Education Act (DSHEA) established legal definitions and label guidelines. It does NOT ensure safety of the product. Always check with a health care professional before taking a supplement. Contact the manufacturer to find out specific amounts of nutrients, botanicals, and herbs. Questions you should ask yourself: Is it safe? Is it effective?

Meet Your Immune System, Bob

Your immune system is your best defense against all the crazy illnesses you come into contact with daily on college campuses. Think of your immune system as your own personal medic. It's always on call, always at the ready, and always there, just for you. But on certain days, your medic is a wreck. I mean, you would be, too, if your boss kept telling you that you had to smoke and to drink and eat unhealthfully. How is this impaired medic

---

SUPPLEMENT SAFETY

Because supplements are still largely unregulated by the federal Food and Drug Administration, it's a good idea to talk with your health care professional before beginning a vitamin/mineral program. Be aware that some doctors and dietitians still do not recognize the myriad benefits of vitamins and minerals, despite numerous studies and hundreds of anecdotal reports that have proven their effectiveness in preserving quality of life. If your doctor or dietitian immediately discounts the idea of a vitamin program, do not be afraid to seek out the opinion of a more progressive practitioner. RealAge.com is a great Web site to look at for science-based evidence to guide your health decisions.

Keep in mind that supplements are highly potent, and you should therefore take every precaution to make sure they will not interact badly with you, each other, or other medications you are taking. Naturopaths and integrative medicine doctors are great expert resources for those looking to start a new vitamin regime.

---

supposed to be your main line of defense? The answer is, he isn't much of one. It's no wonder that people who indulge in these practices are much more likely to suffer from common sicknesses than people who take care of their bodies.

What exactly does your immune system do? Let's give him a name, say, Bob, so you know whom you can thank next time you *don't* catch the head cold both your roommates have. Protecting you from head colds and the like is all in a day's work for good ol' Bob. And that's not all:

➤ Bob determines how fast you age.

➤ Bob fights off viruses, bacteria, and other organisms that try to cause illness (everything from the flu to AIDS).

➤ Bob has the power to destroy cancer cells as they are made.

➤ Bob also serves as your sanitary technician, cleaning out dead cells, dead invaders, and toxic waste products every day.

➤ Bob protects your body from radiation and pollution that could potentially mutate your DNA, causing disease.

➤ If you don't protect him, Bob could deteriorate and make you susceptible to allergies or autoimmune diseases (such as celiac disease).

➤ If Bob is weak, you are ill more frequently, more seriously, and for longer time.

➤ **If Bob is taken care of, he can become the Arnold Schwarzenegger of immune systems, helping you to take on the world.**

SCENARIO 1 Okay, so you wake up in the morning, Bob does his regular check throughout your body for any foreign and possible dangerous entities, and then you sit down for a breakfast of sugary cereal. Bob is starving! Where are his vitamins and minerals? How is he supposed to protect your body, armed with nothing but fat and sugar?

SCENARIO 2 You wake up, Bob checks you out, makes sure you're not dying or anything, and you get right to business, putting away a banana, whole grain cereal, and low-fat yogurt. Yum! Bob is full of potassium, vitamin K, iron, and fiber, ready to take on a day protecting you.

To stay the bodybuilding champion of the world, your immune system needs your help, just as you need his. Vitamin A, B complex, vitamin C, vitamin E, calcium, magnesium, iron, selenium, and zinc are all immune-boosting nutrients. And don't worry—you won't be taking twenty vitamin pills a day. There are plenty of natural food sources for many of these essentials, as well as multivitamins that provide the power of twenty or more vitamins in one or two tablets.

"Aren't Supplements Expensive?"

Some supplements can be expensive, depending on how cost-effective they are to make. Most of the ones you need to take are fairly inexpensive; the more expensive bottles should last you for quite some time. Something you should consider when buying vitamins is that your purchase is an investment. It's more convenient and cheaper to buy a calcium/magnesium pill than to buy enough dairy products to get the same amount of calcium (plus, with most dairy products you are also getting a whole lot of fat and calories). And it's *much* cheaper to get your necessary minerals now than to have to pay an orthopedic surgeon's bill when you're sixty and find you have severe osteoporosis.

"How Do I Know Which Supplements I Need?"

The supplement plan that is right for you depends on your individual needs, which is why it's so crucial for you to see a health care professional and/or a nutritionist before starting on any regimen. The vitamin and mineral plan you start with is a lot like a base car model; it comes only with what you need to drive (live) healthily. You have to specially request air conditioning, radio, heated seats, and 24" rims. With vitamins, you supplement your basic plan with specific nutrients, so that your plan is customized to your needs and wants. For instance, if you develop a cold, for a week or so you'll want to add extra vitamin C and echinacea to your basic plan to help you get over the cold. Later I'll describe a basic plan and discuss what supplements you can add to your regimen for specific ailments.

While some doctors staunchly refute the idea that complementary medicine (such as supplementation with vitamins) is beneficial, most doctors have come to see the huge benefits of combining conventional medicine with alternative therapies. But remember, before you start any supplementary program you should consult with your health care practitioner to make sure that there is no conflict between the vitamins you plan to take and any medication you are currently on, or any known health consideration.

Women between the ages of fifteen and twenty-five can follow the supplement plan below to make sure that all their basic nutritional needs are being met. Your doctor will be able to help you customize a plan for your specific needs. (For instance, if you have a heavy period, your health care practitioner might advise a higher intake of iron than what is generally recommended to replenish your body's supply and stave off any possibility of iron-deficiency anemia.)

BASIC SUPPLEMENT PLAN

1. **MULTIVITAMIN** 1 tablet daily (try Solgar's Formula VM-75 with iron, for menstruating women, or Country Life's Daily Multi-Sorb)

2. **ANTIOXIDANTS: VITAMINS C AND E** Vitamin C with bioflavonoids, 500 milligrams daily (try Natrol's Ester-C or Twinlab's C-Plus Citrus Bioflavonoid Caps); vitamin E, 400 international units (try Twinlab's Super E-Complex, from mixed tocopherols)

3. **MINERALS** You'll get plenty of calcium, magnesium, zinc, and selenium from 2 capsules, 2 times daily of a multimineral vitamin. (Try Twinlab's Cellmins Multi Minerals; also found in multivitamins with minerals.)

4. **ESSENTIAL FATTY ACIDS** 3 softgels daily (try Health from the Sun's Total EFA, or, if you're a vegetarian, try 1 tablespoon of flaxseed oil, either mixed into salad dressing or taken straight)

5. VITAMIN D This is especially important for those of us living north of Atlanta, where sun exposure can be limited. Your body naturally produces enough vitamin D daily from 20 minutes of bright sun exposure (without sunscreen), but for those times of year when you're not able to do this, take 2,500 to 5,000 International Units (IU) of vitamin D (don't worry, it's only about 1 or 2 capsules) to make sure your immune system stays strong. Taking cod liver oil (as I do: 2 teaspoons shaken with a shot of orange juice every morning) is a great way to get vitamin D, since it is a fat-soluble vitamin and needs fat to be absorbed. Otherwise, your body will just excrete it in your urine.

> **VITAMIN 411**
>
> - Unless specified, all supplements should be taken at mealtime.
>
> - The basic plan here includes suggestions of some specific brands. You may choose to use another variety. Be sure to choose high-quality supplements, read the side panel on the bottle or box, and take as directed.
>
> - Supplements are just that: they fill in for deficiencies in your daily diet. They are NOT a substitute for a nutritious diet.

Remember that this is a basic regimen. A dietitian or physician can help you design a more personalized vitamin plan, but this basic recipe is an excellent starting point to help you achieve optimal health. The chart on the next page will give you an idea of the Recommended Daily Allowance of vitamins and minerals.

Recommended Daily Allowance: Vitamins and Minerals

COMPOUND	ADULT FEMALES	COMPOUND	ADULT FEMALES
Vitamin A (daily RE)	800	Iron (Fe) (daily mg)	15
Vitamin D (daily IU)	200	Magnesium (Mg) (daily mg)	320
Vitamin E (daily mg alpha TE)	8	Copper (Cu) (daily mg)	1.5–3
Vitamin K (daily mcg)	65	Zinc (Zn) (daily mg)	12
Vitamin C (daily mg)	60	Selenium (Se) (daily mcg)	55
Folate (daily mcg)	400	Chromium (Cr) (daily mcg)	50–200
Thiamin (B$_1$) (daily mg)	1.1	Molybdenum (Mo) (daily mcg)	75–250
Riboflavin (B$_2$) (daily mg)	1.1	Manganese (Mn) (daily mg)	2–5
Niacin (daily mg)	14	Fluoride (F) (daily mg)	3.0
Pyridoxine (B$_6$) daily mg)	1.3	Sodium (Na) (daily mg)	500
Cyanocobalamine (B$_{12}$) (daily mcg)	2.4	Chloride (Cl) (daily mg)	750
Biotin (daily mcg)	30	Potassium (K) (daily mg)	2,000
Pantothenic Acid (daily mg)	5		
Choline (daily mg)	425		
Calcium (Ca) (daily mg)	1,000		
Phosphorus (P) (daily mg)	700		
Iodine (I) (daily mcg)	150		

g = grams

mg = milligrams (0.001 g)

mcg = micrograms (0.000001 g)

IU = International Units

RE = Retinol Equivalent (1 RE = 3.33 IU vit A or 6 mcg beta carotene)

Alpha TE = Alpha Tocopherol Equivalent

YOU HATE TAKING PILLS, SO EAT YOUR SUPPLEMENTS INSTEAD

You take vitamins to make sure that you still get in pill form any nutrients you are not getting from your food. But I'm sure there will be a few of you who simply can't or won't swallow a pill. Fortunately, all vitamins are derived from natural sources, so I can provide you with a list of a few food items with especially high values of certain vitamins and minerals. That way, you can eat enough of these foods to make sure you have a sufficient daily intake. Another alternative if you simply can't swallow the pills is to try drinking your vitamins. There are a variety of new liquid vitamin drinks that pack a daily dose of vitamins, minerals, and antioxidants into a shot of juice.

All the daily recommendations listed below have been reviewed by dietitians and medical practitioners. If you have any health considerations, however, remember that you should speak with your doctor before making any dietary changes.

Foods High in Calcium

You need about 1,000 milligrams of calcium per day to facilitate weight loss and ensure strong bones, high bone density, and good sleep patterns (since calcium plays a crucial role in muscle relaxation).

MILLIGRAMS PER SERVING

Ricotta cheese, part-skim (1/2 cup)	337
Parmesan cheese (1 ounce)	336
Milk, skim (1 cup)	300
Calcium-fortified orange juice (8 ounces)	263
Yogurt, nonfat (4 ounces)	225
Tofu, firm (1/2 cup)	118
Broccoli (1/2 cup)	89
Chickpeas (1/2 cup)	60

Foods High in Folic Acid
(part of the B-vitamin group)

You need about 400–800 micrograms (mcg) of folic acid daily. Pregnant women especially need folic acid to prevent birth defects in their children. Even before they become pregnant, women should take the recommended daily allowance of folic acid in order to prevent defects in the baby's spine and brain, known as Neural Tube Defects (NTDs). For the rest of us, folic acid is a B vitamin that is used in our bodies for making new cells, and keeping it vibrant.

Remember that vitamins work as a team. This is especially true of B vitamins, which is why you should take a B-complex vitamin as a base and then add specific amounts of certain B vitamins to meet special needs. The Second National Health and Nutrition Examination Survey (NHANES) revealed that 90 percent of women get less than the RDA for vitamin B_6, a type of B vitamin that is essential for the synthesis of serotonin and norepinephrine, two neurotransmitters that are crucial for signaling happy thoughts and emotions in your brain. People who are deficient in this form of B vitamin can experience symptoms such as skin inflammation, depression, confusion, weakness, numbness, and tingling. Basically, think of B vitamins as your energy and mood boosters, and make sure you get plenty!

MILLIGRAMS PER SERVING

Orange juice (1 cup).. 136

Spinach (1/2 cup) 130

Soybeans/edamame (1/2 cup) 100

Asparagus (1/2 cup)... 88

Avocado (1/2 fruit) 81

Lima beans (1/2 cup) 78

Chickpeas (1/2 cup) 70

Sunflower seeds (1 ounce)... 65

Orange sections (1 cup) 54

Broccoli (1/2 cup) 53

Raspberries (1/2 cup) 33

Foods High in Potassium

You need about 2,000–3,000 milligrams of potassium daily to grow, build muscles, transmit nerve impulses throughout your body, and promote healthy heart activity.

MILLIGRAMS PER SERVING

Potato (1 medium)... 844

Cantaloupe (1/2 fruit).. 825

Avocado (1/2 fruit)... 742

Peaches, dried (5 halves) 645

Prunes, dried (10 halves) 626

Tomato juice (1 cup) 536

Yogurt, low-fat (1 cup).. 530

Lima beans (1/2 cup) 517

Salmon (3 ounces) 490

Soybeans/edamame (1/2 cup)... 486

Apricots, dried (10 halves)... 482

Orange juice (1 cup).. 472

Pumpkin seeds (2 ounces)... 458

Sweet potato (1/2 cup) 455

Banana (1 medium) 400

Almonds (2 ounces) 426

Spinach (1/2 cup) 419

Milk, skim (1 cup) 418

Peanuts (2 ounces) 400

Foods High in Selenium

You need about 55 micrograms of selenium daily to prevent cellular damage from free radicals, which may contribute to the development of some cancers and heart disease.

MICROGRAMS PER SERVING

Brazil nuts (about a handful) 544

Sunflower seeds, roasted (about a handful) 78

Tuna (3 ounces) 63

Turkey, light meat (3 ounces) 32

Foods High in Zinc

You need about 15–30 milligrams of zinc daily because it stimulates the production of approximately one hundred enzymes, which are the substances responsible for promoting biochemical reactions in your body. For instance, zinc and the enzymes it stimulates are responsible for a healthy immune system, wound healing, DNA synthesis, and the maintenance of your sense of taste and smell.

MICROGRAMS PER SERVING

Crabmeat (1/2 cup) 6

Turkey, dark meat (3 ounces) 5

Pumpkin and squash seeds (1 ounce) 3

Chicken leg.. 2.7

Yogurt, low-fat, plain (1 cup)..................................... 2.2

Brown rice, cooked (1/2 cup)..................................... 0.6

Baked potato with skin... 0.6

Oatmeal, instant (1/2 cup) 0.6

Beans/Peas 1.5–2

(depending on type)

Foods High in Vitamin C

The Recommended Daily Allowance for vitamin C is 60–75 milligrams, but this is widely accepted as being insufficient. You need about 500 milligrams of vitamin C daily. Because vitamin C cannot be stored in the body—anything you don't use will be flushed out in your urine, so you need to replenish your stock of vitamin C daily. Vitamin C helps body cells, including those in the bones, teeth, gums, and blood vessels, grow and stay healthy. It also helps your body respond to infection and stress, keeping you healthy even when you're struggling to meet deadlines.

MILLIGRAMS PER SERVING

Guava (1 fruit) 165

Red pepper (1 vegetable) 141

Cantaloupe (1/2 fruit)... 113

Green pepper (1 vegetable).. 95

Papaya (1/2 fruit) 94

Strawberries (1 cup) 84

Grapefruit juice (1 cup) 75

Kiwi fruit (1 fruit)... 74

Orange (1 fruit) 70

Orange juice (1/2 cup) 52

Broccoli (1/2 cup cooked or raw)........................49 (cooked), 41 (raw)

Tomatoes (1 cup) 45

Tomato juice (1 cup).. 45

Grapefruit (1/2 fruit) 42

Cauliflower (1/2 cup)... 36

Peas, green, raw (1/2 cup) 31

Foods High in Vitamin D

You need about 600 international units (IU) of vitamin D daily (though everyone in my family takes about 2,500 IU daily and 5,000 daily when we're sick) to maintain normal blood levels of calcium and phosphorous. Vitamin D helps your body to absorb calcium, keeping bones strong; it is also an immune booster. Keep in mind that about twenty minutes of exposure to bright sunlight daily can help you meet your vitamin D needs, but this is hard to do if you live north of Atlanta.

	INTERNATIONAL UNITS
Salmon, pink (3 ounces)	500
Tuna (3 ounces)	200
Milk, skim or 1 percent (8 ounces)	100

Foods High in Vitamin E

You need about 400 IU daily to protect cells in the body from damage caused by free radicals. Free radicals attack cell membranes, proteins, and DNA, and they can ultimately contribute to the development of some cancers and heart disease.

	INTERNATIONAL UNITS (about a handful per serving)
Sunflower seeds	52
Walnuts	22
Almonds	21
Hazelnuts	21
Soybeans, dried	20
Cashews	11
Peanuts, roasted	11
Lima beans, dried	8
Brazil nuts	7
Pecans	2

TWELVE COMMON AILMENTS AND THEIR SUPPLEMENT REMEDIES

College is a pretty safe place. I mean, you have campus security, residential advisers who watch you more closely than your parents did, and friends who stick by you whenever you are coming home from a late-night party across campus. But the fact that you are constantly surrounded by hundreds, maybe even thousands, of people from all over the world means that you are exposed to an infinite number of germs and infections, not to mention coping with menstrual cramps, PMS, yeast infections, and, yes, the occasional hangover. With all these potential hazards in your life, you need all the help you can get, so here are some dietary and supplement remedies for all those common setbacks you thought you had to suffer through like everyone else.

The following are remedies used the world over (and vetted by several MDs) and they have done the trick for me.

1. Common Cold

You know the symptoms. Your throat feels a little scratchy when you wake up. You feel especially warm, even though the heating has been busted for weeks and to everyone else it feels like December in Canada. Your eyes ache, your back aches, you wonder how this could possibly have happened to you. And then you remember that kid who kept sneezing and hacking across the table from you last night at dinner. "Thanks for sharing the wealth, pal," you think gloomily. But then you remember . . . you don't have to suffer through this cold as a commoner would. Just follow this easy recipe and give your immune system (remember good ol' Bob?) the boost it needs to get you over this cold before you can say "Ahhh-choo!"

> ➤ **Vitamin D: 5,000 IU day 1, down to 2,500 until you're recovered. Taking cod liver oil is a great way to get vitamin D, which needs fat to be absorbed (otherwise you just pee it out).**

> ➤ **Vitamin C: Increase intake from 500 to 1000 milligrams daily.**

➤ Echinacea (in capsule, tea, or tincture form): As directed on the label. Try Celestial Seasonings' Echinacea Complete Care Tea or Nature's Herbs' Echinacea Power. You can also try echinacea with added goldenseal, for boosted immune power.

➤ Elderberry extract (in liquid, tea, or capsule form): Use as directed.

➤ Zinc (lozenges): Take with food.

2. Sore Throat

This common malady sometimes accompanies your cold or comes on its own, especially when you aren't getting enough sleep or are sleeping in a very dry room. Drugstore-variety throat lozenges, especially those with lemon and honey, are very helpful for mild soreness. Also, drinking tea with honey and lemon can help. But when you need something with a little more kick to get over a sore throat, try the following tried-and-true remedies:

➤ Mix $1/2$ teaspoon of salt into one cup of warm water and add Weleda Ratanhia Mouthwash with myrrh (as directed on bottle) to the solution. Gargle for thirty seconds and spit. Repeat until solution is finished. Do not rinse; you want the solution to coat your throat and stay there as long as possible, so that the beneficial properties of the salt and myrrh have the most time to work.

➤ Pour five to ten drops of NutriBiotic's Grapefruit Seed Extract into one cup of warm water and gargle for sixty seconds.

➤ Drink tea as often as you like. Two that are especially useful for curing sore throats are Celestial Seasonings' Throat Soothers and Traditional Medicinals' Throat Coat.

➤ Warm chicken soup or miso soup (clear, warm liquids) also help soothe the pain associated with sore throats.

3. Nausea and Stomachache

Determining the cause of your nausea is the first step to curing it. It could be that you ate some bad fried sole in the dining hall last night, or maybe you ate too much in general and are feeling a bit bloated. Being overtired can also lead to nausea, as can gas buildup in your stomach. Drinking ginger or mint tea can help ease mild nausea. I love Celestial Seasonings' Tummy Mint tea for mild stomach discomfort or even just as a palate cleanser after a meal. Bubbly drinks, especially ginger ale (since it has the added bonus of nausea-calming ginger), can be very useful for breaking up stubborn gas in the stomach to help ease nausea. Just be sure to opt for a natural or health-food-store version of whatever bubbly drink you choose so you avoid the high-fructose corn syrup most conventional sodas use as sweetener. If you actually do have food poisoning, however, you may require a physician's attention. You'll need to keep well hydrated with liquids like Gatorade that replenish not only water but also the salts and sugars that you lose when you have diarrhea, to keep from becoming dehydrated. Most health food stores have a natural electrolyte drink, free from all the unnecessary color and sugar additives, though Gatorade works in a pinch. If you have diarrhea more than four times a day for more than a day, you should see a doctor. Unfortunately, all the natural remedies in the world won't help you get over a bingefest—you'll just have to wait out that sick feeling and maybe this brief time of suffering will keep you from repeating the mistake.

4. PMS and Cramps

Menstrual cramps—those horrible aches in your lower abdomen, back, and even your thighs—are created by prostaglandins, chemicals your body releases at the start of your period signaling your uterus to contract and push out its old lining. Every woman's body makes different amounts of these chemicals, and the more you produce the harder your contractions and the more painful your cramps. Luckily, there are ways to make the muscle contractions hurt less.

➤ **Always take your calcium. Calcium relaxes your muscles, like the ones that seize up when you experience cramps. Eating calcium-rich foods, such as milk and yogurt, each day (not just during your period) will lessen the severity of cramps and food cravings.**

➤ **Magnesium, along with vitamin B$_6$, will help with the anxiety, irritability, and mood swings that can be part of PMS, so during that time of the month add two capsules daily of Twinlab's Calcium Citrate plus magnesium to your Twinlab's Multi Mineral dosage (four capsules daily). High doses of magnesium may cause diarrhea in some** individuals; if this occurs, lessen the dose. Magnesium plays an important role in metabolic processes needed for exercise and protein synthesis. Clinical signs of magnesium deficiency include muscle spasms.

Aside from taking supplements, there are other things you can do to reduce cramping:

➤ Avoid caffeine, alcohol, and nicotine. These stimulants will encourage your muscles to contract more frequently and with stronger force. Plus, who feels like having a shot or brew when there are shooting pains in your abdomen?

➤ Get plenty of exercise. This is not only important for weight loss. Thirty minutes of exercise three times a week keeps the flow of blood and oxygen strong, so that your contractions won't be as painful. Go for a jog or a swim. I know this sounds like the last thing you'd want to do when you're doubled over with cramps, but it will make your body release endorphins, those "happy" chemicals, which will ease the pain fast.

➤ Get to sleep. An all-night party is okay once in a while, but at college you may find that once in a while means every weekend. But it is important, especially for menstruating females, to get enough sleep, since a well-rested body is better able to tolerate pain (so cramps won't feel as bad to you).

➤ Omega-3 fats. Eating one serving twice a week of fatty fish (such as salmon or tuna) or some nuts (also high in omega-3s) or flaxseeds will help your body control its output of prostaglandins.

➤ Heat is the best remedy. Soak in a hot bath for ten minutes (if one isn't available, try the whirlpool at the sports complex). Keep an electric heating pad under your bed, and use it to heat your abdomen and help blood flow to that area. Sipping hot tea such as Traditional Medicinals' PMS Tea will also help ease the pain. You can also use other caffeine-free herbal teas, which help increase blood flow to the cramp region and reduce the pain and frequency.

5. Headache

Again, you may need to be your own doctor in determining how you got your headache. If it is a mild tension headache, a little rest and some deep breathing may be all you need. If it is coming from a stiff neck, get a room-mate to rub your neck or do it yourself to stretch out the neck muscles and release pressure from the back of your brain. Many headaches are caused by low blood sugar, so, if you haven't eaten in a while, grab a fruit or some other food that will deliver sugar to your blood but won't spike your insulin output (a candy bar is not the answer). If you think your headache is related to a more serious illness, see a doctor.

Migraine headaches, shooting pains in the back of the neck or forehead, respond well to magnesium and coenzyme Q_{10} (CoQ_{10}) taken daily. Try 400 milligrams of magnesium citrate and 60 milligrams of CoQ_{10} twice daily.

6. Sore Muscles and Minor Sprains

Playing three varsity sports definitely takes its toll on the body. I played tennis, basketball, and lacrosse throughout high school and have experienced my fair share of sore muscles, sprained ankles, and tender tendons. Taking arnica Montana, a homeopathic remedy for swelling, bruising, minor sprains and strains, and muscle soreness, immediately after an injury really helped get me through the seasons. Arnica can be taken in pill form dissolved under the tongue (it tastes like sugar) or it can be applied directly as a cream (if the skin is not broken). You can pick up arnica at most pharmacies or health food stores. Follow the directions on the label, as the strength of the product you choose will affect the dosage. For an acute sprain or strain, take 30X potency, as directed. For a chronic problem, take 6X or 9X as directed. Cease after symptoms subside or after two weeks.

Also, bromelain (derived from pineapples) is a natural anti-inflammatory. In fact, plastic surgeons have begun to prescribe it to their nose-job patients for a dramatically faster recovery and less noticeable bruising. Even if you don't plan on altering your nose, bromelain can help you heal more quickly from any sort of bruising or inflammation. Take 250 to 500 milligrams (i.e., Twinlab's Mega Bromelain), three times daily, away from meals.

7. Fatigue

Many college students suffer from what they think is fatigue, but is more likely inertia resulting from poor eating habits and lack of exercise. Diet can greatly affect your energy level, so make sure you are getting all your nutritional requirements. Also, and this may sound contradictory, when you are fatigued during the day, it is extremely important to exercise;

this will keep up your energy levels, so you can still function. If you find yourself falling asleep in class, ask to go to the bathroom and then do a few jumping jacks and stretches in the hallway to get the blood flowing throughout your body. If you must stay in class, concentrate on regular, deep breathing and tap your foot or perform some other small movement to get your blood flowing. Then, when you have time, head to the gym for a short workout.

Some students actually do suffer from unusual lethargy, tiredness, and lack of energy without any apparent cause. The onset of such fatigue may be an early sign of illness. If you have sudden, unexplained fatigue, you should see a doctor immediately so he or she can run tests to rule out the possibility of any serious ailment, such as iron-deficiency anemia or mononucleosis.

In most cases, you will not have a serious illness. Remember that depression, anxiety, and stress—which you may experience during your adjustment from home to college life—all bring your energy level down. Sleep habits are never great at college, but try to get seven to eight hours of good-quality sleep a night or you may put your body at serious risk for infection and illness, not to mention looking a bit haggard. Make sure you find some balance between your social and academic lives so that you have time to sleep. A few too many nights out with friends is all you need to send you over the edge into zombieland.

8. Insomnia

Drinking caffeinated beverages, watching scary or thrilling movies, or listening to upbeat music right before going to bed are surefire ways to guarantee you'll be lying awake an hour later. Right before bed, try some relaxation time, during which you concentrate on breathing regularly and deeply, listen to calming music, pray, meditate, and take time to clear your mind of worries that will distract you as you try to get to sleep. You can also sip some Celestial Seasonings Sleepytime, or Sleepytime Extra (with valerian), while reading in bed to put you in the mood for sleep. Also, take four capsules of Twinlab's Calcium Citrate plus magnesium before bedtime; if you are taking the Multi Minerals, reduce these to two a day while you are taking the Calcium Citrate. As long as you're not going above the Recommended Daily Allowance of calcium (unless specified to do so by your physician), extra calcium and magnesium should help your muscles relax, which will help you fall asleep, without any side effects.

9. Urinary Tract Infection (UTI)

A urinary tract infection is caused by bacteria and is generally treated with antibiotics, which you will need to get from a doctor. There are some things you can do to guard against it. When sharing a communal toilet, don't sit on the seat or, if you must, clean it with a sanitizer first. To protect yourself against infection, or if you already have a UTI, you can speed the healing process by drinking plenty of filtered or spring water (at least eight 12-ounce glasses a day to flush out the toxins circulating in your body). Also, drinking 100 percent cranberry juice, not cranberry cocktail (sweetened with high-fructose corn syrup) will help eliminate the damaging bacteria. You can also take cranberry capsules from Nature's Herbs as directed on the product label.

10. Yeast Infection, or Vaginitis

A diet rich in acidophilus—a bacteria found in yogurt with live cultures that promotes vaginal health—and free of yeast-based foods (such as bread) is the first step to keeping yourself free of yeast infections. As always, drink plenty of filtered or spring water. And, should you choose to supplement, you can use 50 milligrams of Twinlab's Super B Complex (one capsule, once daily) and Nature's Way Primadophilus (one capsule daily, or as instructed by your doctor) or a powerful probiotic like lactobacillus acidophilus, as directed on the label.

11. Constipation

Occasional constipation is most likely due to a lack of fiber and water in your diet. Ideally you want your poop to look like a banana, pretty much the shape of your large intestine, since this means you have had a complete bowel movement. (What do you want from me? We're talking about constipation . . . it has to be a little gross.) To counteract a constipation problem, increase your fiber intake by eating plenty of whole, fresh fruit and vegetables; bran cereals; whole grains, such as brown rice and oatmeal; and prunes or prune juice. You can also add one tablespoon of ground flaxseeds to cereal, yogurt, soup, or salads for added fiber. You can also take a dietary supplement such as Metamucil (psyllium husks) to ensure that you are getting enough fiber. You'd be surprised how much a difference it can make simply to start each day with a bowl of high-fiber, high-protein, healthful cereal and to eat salads.

> ➤ **Increase your liquid intake. Drink eight 12-ounce glasses of water daily in addition to other liquids. This will lubricate your system.**

> ➤ **Aloe vera juice (not gel!) soothes the intestines when ingested. Follow the directions on the bottle to be sure**

that you don't give yourself too much soothing power and send yourself over to the other side of the bowel movement spectrum.

➤ If you're not getting anywhere with simple dietary changes, Metamucil powder (i.e., psyllium husks) is a great source of fiber, mixed into a liquid (like a smoothie). This can be found at your local drugstore or health food shop.

➤ If you suffer from prolonged, painful constipation, your problem may be more serious and you should consult your doctor immediately.

12. Diarrhea

You get diarrhea when the beneficial bacteria in your intestines die because of an infection or virus; consequently, there is no "flora and fauna" to . . . well, hold your poop together. To resuscitate these bacteria, you need to drink sugar water, in the form of apple juice (or some other juice, if apple isn't your fave). You should be drinking plenty of fluids, especially those with electrolytes and sugars (natural versions of ginger ale and Gatorade), to keep yourself hydrated, since you will be losing lots of fluid and minerals in your poop. Once you've provided the bacteria with its basic food (sugar), you need to get some bread and rice into your system to soak up the excess liquids and help give your feces some form. Pretty gross, huh? No more gross than having diarrhea, though. And finally, tea, the magic cure for just about anything, has many healing powers and may just make you feel better. Put these four key words together and you get the mnemonic B.R.A.T.: Bread, Rice, Apple Juice, Tea. That's easy to remember.

You can also take lactobacillus acidophilus/bifidus as directed on the label—the probiotic we talked about earlier that helps keep your digestive system in working order.

If you are suffering from a serious illness and you have diarrhea more than four times daily for more than a day, see a physician.

I'll bet by this time you know more about supplements than you ever dreamed possible. Feel free to share your new wealth of information by teaching your friends (or even your parents) about the benefits supplements and natural remedies can have. (But remember that other people may need drastically different doses of certain vitamins than you do.)

Helping your body stay healthy and strong physically is so important, but so is making sure that you are emotionally healthy, too. And this brings us to our next step: living an enlightened life of peace, serenity, and service.

STEP 8

GET HAPPY

*A More Relaxed,
More Effective You*

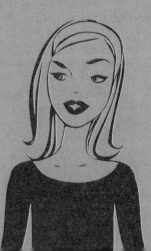

S O NOW YOU know how to eat healthfully, squeeze exercise into even the most hectic of schedules, and even how to supplement your new healthy lifestyle with vitamins and minerals. You would think that all this would be enough to get you through life—or at least through the next round of finals. But it's been my experience that even the most healthful, athletic, well-supplemented individuals sometimes need a chance to relax and rejuvenate.

College life presents us with so many idiots who drive us nuts—no, that's not right. College life gives us so many useless assignments—no, that's not it, either. Ah, got it. College life presents us with so many opportunities for struggle and growth, but almost no opportunities to calm down. We're all so busy running around from classes to dorm, dorm to gym, gym to dorm, dorm to party, party to party, party to dorm, it seems that if we want a chance to relax, we'd better start looking for the twenty-fifth hour in the day. This pace can drive us to use food, especially unhealthy food, for comfort, rather than finding other ways to cope.

Food is for fuel; breathing and meditation are for comfort.

Fortunately, relaxing and de-stressing do not have to take up huge amounts of time. They are free, health-enhancing practices that can totally change your outlook on life by making you more open to change and more accepting of yourself.

WHY WE NEED TO DE-STRESS: COPING WITH FIGHT OR FLIGHT

When you experience a stressful event, your brain releases chemicals into your bloodstream to help your body cope with the anxiety and fear that result from a perceived threat. Adrenaline is one of those chemicals. When it is released, your body goes into high gear, preparing to deal with the potential danger. This reflexive reaction to stress is known as fight or flight, since our instinctual response to danger is either to engage in battle, or to split. This response is triggered not only when a lion is about to pounce on you, as some of our ancestors experienced. Being anxious about a final exam, an oral presentation, or walking into yet another roomful of unfamiliar faces is enough to set off alarms of danger in our bodies. The muscles in your neck, shoulders, and face may stiffen, creating a kind of internal armor. You may notice your heart racing, your body temperature increasing, your hands getting clammy, or your breath becoming short. These are signs that your body is preparing itself to fight—or to run for its life.

Eventually, in order to cope with the increased stress, your body will shut off those functions that are not completely essential to your survival in an emergency. So, for instance, your immune system might be temporarily closed down, since it is not critical to fighting or fleeing. (Sorry, Bob.) This is why people who are constantly under stress are more likely to get sick. Over time, the body gets tired from constantly preparing to fight with, or run from, perceived threats. Unless you find a way to get rid of the stress, or cope with it better, you can seriously compromise your health. Your body doesn't get sick leave or paid vacations, so you need to find other ways to give it a break. In the rest of this chapter, I'll discuss some of those ways.

BREATHING

We take for granted that our body is programmed to breathe automatically, and we stop thinking about the actions involved: inhaling and exhaling. We derive our life force from breathing. Try consciously inhaling five deep breaths and exhaling five deep breaths. You'll be amazed how much more oxygen you take in when you focus on breathing than when you perform this action on autopilot. This extra oxygen courses throughout your body, from your brain, to your heart, to your toes, refueling every cell and increasing your energy production by oxygenating the mitochondria. The mitochondria are the organelles in each cell that take fuels such as proteins and fats and burn them to drive cellular processes, like cell renewal. And when you consciously and fully exhale, you pump out a much greater amount of carbon dioxide, cleansing your body of this toxic gas. You can use your ability to regulate your oxygen intake and your carbon dioxide output to help energize yourself and relax. The following example is only one of millions of situations in which breathing can make the difference between feeling helpless or feeling empowered.

Say you just got home after taking your molecular biology final. You spent thirty-six hours looking over almost every page in your more than two-thousand-page text. You thought you knew everything any humane professor could possibly expect you to know for a final, but, to your dismay, your professor is anything but. The one topic you thought you were safe skimming over turned out to be the central theme of the exam, and you want to kick yourself for not having seen it coming. Now you're back in your dorm, imagining the look on your parents' faces as they lay on the guilt trip: "I can't believe you got an F! Did you study at all?" Worst of all, you have an even harder exam tomorrow that you didn't study for because of molecular biology, and now you're in such a rotten state of mind that you might as well not study, since even thirty-six hours of studying is clearly not enough.

Unfortunately, all the moping and self-flagellation in the world won't spare you an F (if that is, indeed, what you scored) *after* you've taken the test. True, it may be your fault that you didn't leave yourself enough time to study for tomorrow's exam, but that decision is in the past. The best thing to do now is to approach your next task with a clear, relaxed mind. Dwelling on something that you cannot change only saps your energy. I know everyone likes to, and maybe even needs to, play a little self-pity ditty on that violin. But when you realize how silly this tactic is, try a short breathing exercise (like the one that follows) to help you relax, let go of what's already done, and get back on track.

FIND A PLACE WHERE roommates, friends, phone calls, e-mail, or any other outside distractions won't bother you. Close your eyes and visualize your favorite, most relaxing spot. Maybe a sandy strip of deserted beach, a cozy chair next to a fire, a snowy slope, or a lovely trail through the woods. Place yourself in a door looking out on your relaxing spot of choice. Now, before you step through the door and begin to relax, visualize each of your worries stacked neatly on your left. Imagine giving the neat pile a good kick, scattering your worries in every direction. Next, step though the door and enter your relaxing world. Begin to focus only on your breath. Breathe in and out five times, deeply and slowly.

With each breath in, imagine yourself inhaling that sweet, tropical air, or that clear mountain freshness. See this rejuvenation coursing through your entire body, cleansing it of any remaining emotional and mental baggage. Then, as you breathe out, cleanse yourself of all this weight. With each breath, feel your lungs expand and contract in strong, consistent, powerful motion. See yourself glowing inside and out from all the clean air pumping through your now weightless body. A dark spot on your glowing body represents any place where tension still exists. Focus on that spot and feel your breath immediately become more active in that area, cleansing and purifying that part and making it glow like the rest of you. Now you should feel energy and warmth filling your entire body, replacing the cold of anger, depression, and fatigue.

Once you feel you have been thoroughly cleansed, start to familiarize yourself again with the surrounding world. Hear the sounds, feel the temperature, and realize how you are a part of this place. Collect your scattered concerns and replace them in your refreshed, relaxed, and energized mind. You now have power and control, where before there was helplessness and despair. You have control over your inner life and how you react to the events of your external environment. You can deal with anything in your path, just as long as you remember to use your breathing for energy and relaxation.

Breathing need not be used only as a coping measure when you are depressed, angry, or despairing. You can use breathing to head off these symptoms before they start. For instance, use deep, conscious breathing to increase your energy if you start getting sleepy in the middle of studying. That way, you won't have to skim the section that ends up being the main focus of your exam. Or breathe for relaxation right before your exam, when you feel a wave of panic coming on, so that whatever information you did study stays clear and accessible in your mind. You may not have control over the actions of others or over the obstacles that appear in your life path; the only thing you can control is your response to these events. Prepare yourself to respond in the best way possible by breathing fully and staying relaxed.

MEDITATION

Meditation can be as simple as just a few spare moments spent in silence. It does not have to be an elaborate process during which you achieve spiritual enlightenment. The point of meditation is to help you quiet your mind, and to notice how you react to the thoughts and feelings that inevitably pass through your mind while you are trying to be quiet. Meditation helps you bring your consciousness back to the present. We spend so much time thinking about our futures or our pasts, what we'll be doing tomorrow or what we screwed up yesterday. It's so much more important for us to be present in and engaged with this day, this moment, first. So, while meditation can help you get more out of the future, its main purpose is to help you live within the present.

Meditation sometimes involves sitting still in a certain position for a period of time and focusing on your breathing. You may prefer to do a walking meditation, quieting your mind as you move without speaking through the countryside, or the streets of your neighborhood.

Meditation can be hard in the beginning, since you're attempting to let go of the thoughts that occupy you, to give yourself a blissful break from worrying. It makes you realize how often our thoughts are controlling us, rather than the other way around! There are plenty of good books and manuals available to help you begin a meditation practice. One of the best is *Wherever You Go, There You Are: Mindfulness Meditation in Everyday Life,* by Jon Kabat-Zinn. You may even want to find a class or seminar near your college campus, since an instructor might be able to answer many of your questions, and meditation is often even more effective when done in a group.

After you've meditated a little bit, you may find that you've reached a new level of calm that can help you work through any problems or stresses in your life. Find a quiet place to sit, stand, or lie down for a few minutes. Allow your mind to relax and then single out each of the things that are pressing on your mind, making you anxious, uncomfortable, angry, or sad. With practice, you may be surprised at your ability to pinpoint the source of your depression or anxiety when you take a calm moment to reflect. Once you've discovered the issues that are bothering you, evaluate them to see if you have control over them or if they depend on the actions of others. If it turns out that you have no control over the situation, you need to recognize this fact and realize that there is nothing to be gained from fretting over such an issue. This can be very difficult, as you naturally want to be able to control the actions of others, or at least want to have complete control over the events of your own life. But the fact is that you do not. Bossy as you may be, no one has to do exactly as you tell him or her to, nor does the weather have to obey you, nor will you be able to avoid mishaps in your life. Accept these facts and stop wasting valuable energy trying to control things that cannot be controlled. If, however, you do have control over whatever is bothering you, then you need to decide how you want to deal with the situation. Keep in mind that you may not be able to solve all your problems in one sitting.

MASSAGE AND REFLEXOLOGY

I have never met someone who did not like a good rubdown. I'm talking about a body massage that works out the tension in each of your muscles, leaving you completely rested and limber.

Massages relax muscles by helping eliminate lactic acid, which is one of the by-products of muscle work. A full body massage helps improve circulation, as well as your lymphatic system, the part of your immune system that does maintenance work on your body, such as carrying toxins away from your muscles. (This is why it is so important for you to drink lots of water before and after a massage—to flush out all the toxins that are being released through the kneading of your muscles.) I don't think I need to spend any more time convincing you how great a massage can be, whether just to relax and rejuvenate, or as therapy after an injury. I will mention that professional massage therapists have in-depth knowledge of each of the primary muscle groups, how they are connected, and how to relieve tension in each of these sore spots. Some of them are even trained in reflexology, a form of bodywork that correlates external points on the soles of the feet with various internal organs and processes. Pressing on these different foot points is supposed to stimulate healthy functioning inside the body. Reflexology bases some of its practices on principles rooted in traditional Chinese medicine, whereby using pressure points around the body to stimulate the flow of energy can help heal and promote optimal health. But reflexology practitioners can have hourly rates that end in multiple zeros—out of reach for the typical college student. What you may not realize is that anyone you know is a massage therapist waiting to be trained . . . by you. That's right, trading massages with your roommates, your boyfriend—just about anyone—is a great way to get a free massage, not to mention boost your popularity (trust me, they'll be flocking to you).

HEAVEN SCENT: AROMATHERAPY

Aromatherapy is defined as the use of volatile plant oils, including essential oils (those oils that give plants their characteristic scent), for psychological and physical well-being. This pretty much means that you use different scents to soothe, calm, or energize yourself. Different scents can have significant effects on the body, from putting you to sleep, to waking you up, to clearing up congestion—even increasing your sex drive. It's all about knowing which scents do what for you.

Essential oils are made up of tiny molecules that dissolve easily in alcohol, skin creams, and oils (fats). In these mediums, essential oils can quickly penetrate the skin and permeate the entire body by mixing with the fat tissue below the skin. In addition, as the oil molecules evaporate from the skin's surface, they are inhaled, sending messages straight to the brain via the millions of sensitive cells in your nose. These inhaled molecules affect your emotions by working on the portion of your brain called the limbic system, which, coincidentally, also controls the major functions of the body, such as sleep, sex drive, hunger, and thirst. The limbic system also governs memory, which explains why there is such a strong link between smell and memory. Every time you smell something, whether it's fresh-baked bread or dog droppings, your brain immediately reacts and tells the rest of your body what to do. That direction could be to relax and calm down, or to start checking the bottoms of your shoes. If your sense of smell can have such a dramatic influence on your mood and level of stress, why not learn how to harness that power for good?

You can do this by using essential oils. My favorite way is to place a bowl with a few drops of essential oils in it on my desk or next to my bed to immediately rejuvenate or relax me. Placing it over a heat source will help the oils evaporate even more quickly. There are plenty of other ways to use essential oils. You can use them in conjunction with other oils to give yourself a nice body rub. To do this, simply add three to five drops of an essential oil to two teaspoons of a carrier oil. A carrier oil is a vegetable oil that is used to dilute the essential oil. Some examples that you can easily find in a supermarket or health food store are almond oil, carrot oil, evening primrose oil, grapeseed oil, jojoba oil, olive oil, peanut oil, sesame oil, and sunflower oil. Always go for cold-pressed, unrefined, certified organic oil whenever possible to get the most essential fatty acids and vitamins. (The less refined the oil is, the darker it will be.) You can choose which essential oils you want to smell like after your massage, though certain scents have been linked to different effects. For instance, lavender is calming; citrus is enlivening; eucalyptus is cleansing; and jasmine is intoxicating (puts you in the mood, so to speak). Health food stores such as Whole Foods, Trader Joe's, or Wild Oats all carry a variety of essential oils with explanations of what their scents promise to do for you. Pick your own!

But essential oils aren't good only for massage. If you can boil water, you can create a great aromatic steam. Use five drops of a peppermint or eucalyptus essential oil per liter of boiling water to ease a cold or sinus congestion, or just two drops per liter for a gentler relaxing effect on the nasal passages. Pour the mixture into a large bowl or sink, lean over the bowl, and place a towel over your head and shoulders to lock in the steam. Voilà!

You can also use essential oils in compresses for muscle sprains or bruises. Simply soak a towel in a bowl with three to four drops of lavender oil added per every 8 ounces of hot or cold water and fix firmly on the hurt spot. Use cold water for bruising, swelling, or inflammation. Use hot water for older injuries where there isn't swelling or inflammation. You should generally consult a physician for any serious injury, but these compresses can help with the milder ones. All of us know what a long day can do to feet and hands; soaking tired hands and feet in warm water with essential oils can help. The warmth of the water used to soak your hands or feet helps your blood vessels dilate, which can also help alleviate tension headaches caused by blood vessels in the head becoming engorged with blood. Try a foot soak next time you have a pounding headache and see if you don't feel better in a jiffy.

If nothing is wrong with you physically, but you feel a little down emotionally, you can use essential oils simply to boost your mood—citrus scents are especially good for this purpose. Just add a few drops of oil to a bowl of water and allow the oil to evaporate and fill your dorm room (or any other space) with a lovely aroma. You can also purchase a diffuser or a ceramic heat ring, both of which are affixed to a lightbulb to heat the oil and speed up the evaporation process. Various aroma combinations and diffusing contraptions can be found at health food stores.

Essential oils can also help you retain that ridiculous amount of calculus you've been cramming into your brain for tomorrow's final. And no, it's not because certain oils can alter your gray matter and turn you into Einstein. But they can unlock mental blocks that might be keeping you from memorizing efficiently. Peppermint oil has been shown to be effective in enhancing memory, and you can blend this scent with orange or lemon to make the mix invigorating and stimulating.

Oils can also help in the love department. Certain scents, like pumpkin pie, vanilla, and cinnamon, are most attractive to men. (So that's why guys love Thanksgiving so much—and you thought it was the football games!) Lavender, licorice, and vanilla are the most attractive scents to women. Jasmine and rose, the king and queen of essential oils, respectively, are attractive to just about anyone. So dab a bit of these scents on as a perfume, or add a few drops of oil to your body cream, to make a natural aphrodisiac that's sure to attract everyone for miles around.

Sometimes you may want to mix more than one scent. When you blend scents, the oils combine and a new compound is formed that has slightly different properties than the individual oils. When combining oils, you want to act like a perfumer: you need to pay attention to top, middle, and base notes. Fresh scents, such as lemon, eucalyptus, or tea tree, are top notes, which are generally fresh, light, and immediately detectable because of their high evaporation rate. Floral oils and the softer herbs, including lavender, geranium, chamomile, and peppermint, make up most of the middle notes, the heart of the mixture, and are detectable after the top note, when smelling the scent for the first time. Wood oils such as frankincense and sandalwood form the base notes, which are rich, heavy odors that linger and emerge fully only after being exposed to the air for a prolonged time. Of course, there are a few exceptions. For instance, jasmine and rose are floral scents that fall into the base notes category. A good blend will combine one oil from each of these three categories, usually in this proportion: three drops top note, two drops of middle note, and two drops of the base note. You can, of course, go totally wild and crazy and have two middle notes and a base note, or a top note and a base note and no middle note. Go with what your inner Coco Chanel tells you, and let your nose be your guide.

Below you'll find a brief list of moods and the scents that enhance them, as well as different ways to use aromatherapy with diffusers.

UPLIFTING, ENERGIZING **lemon, tangerine, grapefruit, strawberry**

RELAXING, SOOTHING **chamomile, lavender, vanilla**

SENSUAL **ylang-ylang, musk, jasmine**

DECONGESTING **eucalyptus, peppermint**

MOST ATTRACTIVE TO MEN **pumpkin pie, vanilla, cinnamon**

MOST ATTRACTIVE TO WOMEN **licorice, vanilla, lavender**

FAITH AND MEANING

My family is pretty religious. And, like many other teenagers, I went through a period during which religion was number one billion on my list of things to care about. Honestly, what could I possibly have to gain from going to church every Sunday? I'd already heard all the Bible stories. How many times can you hear the Christmas story retold? Religion just didn't do it for me anymore.

One day I calmly suggested to my parents that I be exempted from the family's Sunday church trips. As you can imagine, this didn't go over too well. I was forced to go to church nearly every Sunday until I left for college. There really wasn't anything I could do about it, stubborn though I was (and am!). What was I supposed to say? "Religion is bad for me— that's why I don't want to go." Even I couldn't say this with much conviction. The truth was, it was more being forced to do something, to believe in something—than the actual hour spent in church each Sunday—that made me feel trapped and gave me the negative feelings I began to associate with church, God, and organized religion altogether.

Okay. So cut to my first year in college. No one was forcing me to go to church! I didn't even have to think about anything to do with religion if I didn't want to. All ecclesiastical words were completely erased from my vocabulary. And you know what? I was really happy. I was happy that I didn't have to obey my parents. I was happy that I didn't have to worship anyone. I was happy that I did not have to wake up early on Sunday mornings. These are all completely normal feelings for a teenager to have. But I came to see that religion served more of a purpose in my life than I had once believed, and regretted not having it as a presence. Part of being a young adult in college is having the freedom to make mistakes, and, you hope, the intelligence to learn from them.

As the school year wore on, more and more I found that my life lacked something; I didn't have any concept of a higher purpose or duty. Going to church had been my primary source of learning about something outside of myself. I'm not just talking about memorizing the Ten Commandments or remembering to treat others as you want to be treated. In my religion, much of the biblical interpretation has to do with finding your higher purpose, discovering why you are on Earth.

As a teenager, it's fun and easy to assume that you are living primarily to serve yourself. But in college, I learned that happiness and self-confidence do not come from having everyone tell you how wonderful you are, but from showing yourself that you can serve others. While all along I had credited religion with being the source of my unhappiness, resentment, and discomfort, in reality I was the source of my unhappiness, resentment, and discomfort. Once I realized this, religion no longer posed the threat it once had. I started attending chapel services at my college infrequently and found that even these small doses of prayer and contemplation really gave me a centeredness and focus away from me, me, me, me, me.

It doesn't matter what religion you are, or even if you believe in God at all. You can still understand the good feeling that comes from being a useful human being in the world. What are we here on Earth for if not to help one another to make it a better place? It takes time to get used to putting other people ahead of yourself, but now that you're in college and are becoming an adult (and want to be treated like one), it's time not only to grow older, but to grow up.

STEP 9

GET CONSCIOUS

Food for Thought

WHEN YOU SIT down to a meal, whether in the dining hall, on your dorm room floor, at a restaurant, or even at home, do you ever wonder how the food you're about to eat got to you? Where was it grown and how? Was it produced organically, or with the help of pesticides and fertilizers? Did it come from a farm the next town over, or from a greenhouse in Chile? Ultimately, will this food help or hurt your body, and how will it affect the environment?

These are questions every "conscious eater" must ask herself when making the decision of what to eat. Why? Well, because not all foods are created equal. If you're eating strawberries in December and go to school in the Northeast, chances are they were grown several thousand miles away, maybe even in another country, and were exposed to pesticides, fertilizers, and preservatives so that they would grow round and red (though not necessarily sweet or delicious) and appear fresh when they arrive all the way back on your plate. These days, more and more boxed breakfast items, such as cereal and toaster strudel, claim to be made from "whole grains." But there are generally very few visible kernels of fibrous goodness

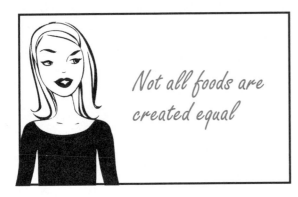

Not all foods are created equal

in these convenience meals, and a whole lot of invisible high-fructose corn syrup, sugar's cheaper—and more toxic—substitute. The more you know about what is *actually* in your food, the harder it is to make poor choices.

THE PRICE GAP

One of the first things I noticed when I started food shopping for myself was how expensive healthy food can be. Even between a conventional item and its organic version, the price gap can be astounding! As I began to look over my receipts and peruse the aisles of my local grocery and health food stores, I noticed an obvious (and disturbing) trend: The more heavily processed and artificial a food, the less expensive it was.

How is it that something that you eat exactly the way it looks when it comes out of the ground or off a tree can cost more than something that went through a day and a half of mechanical digestion by heavy machinery? Doesn't it strike you as a bit odd that our supermarkets are crammed with 99-cent bags of chips, but apples can cost $1.25 or more? Or that a hamburger at a fast-food restaurant might run just under $4 compared to a large salad that can cost twice that?

This got me thinking: What is it about our food system that makes it easier (and more profitable) to produce fake junk foods? I started digging a little deeper and began to uncover the principles and players at the core of our current food system. I'm sad to say it's not a very pretty picture. While here in America we are very fortunate to have an abundance of things we can eat, these "foods" bear little resemblance to those that would support our health and sustain us for the long term.

Collectively, we spend a lot more money on health care than we do on food, but there seems to be an interesting correlation between how much cheap, processed food people eat (proportional to the rest of their diet) and how much money they end up needing to spend for health care later on down the line. It sounds like it would probably just be easier to get more healthy foods on the table to begin with and avoid all the chronic illness. So what's the holdup?

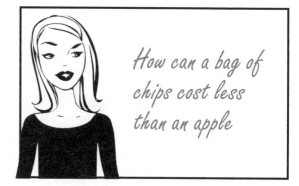

How can a bag of chips cost less than an apple

SUBSIDIES

In sum, it has become too hard to be healthy in America largely because it is so expensive to purchase good food. Subsidies are one of the major reasons for this disparity in price between wholesome options and their junk-food counterparts.

Look at the example of a hamburger at a fast-food restaurant. First, you have the beef, which involves raising and slaughtering livestock, processing the meat, potentially freezing it, and shipping it to the point of sale. Then you have the bun that is made of processed flour, which means that all the wheat had to be grown, harvested, ground, mixed, baked and then shipped. In addition, there are whatever vegetables and spreads might be included. You get all this for $4 but if you want to eat a head of lettuce and some dressing it's going to cost you twice the amount?! How can this be?

Back in the early 1900s, the U.S. government invested in an agriculture policy that aimed to promote production of those foods that could be easily stored or shipped to soldiers fighting in World War I, such as corn and wheat. To make sure we had plenty of these grains, we decided to pay farmers to grow more of the crops we needed most—and consequently stop growing other grains, vegetables, and fruits. This practice is what we know as *subsidizing*. Today, we spend more than $25 billion in subsidies to support farmers of corn, wheat, soybeans, canola, cows and dairy products, chickens, and pigs.

Because this government money was used to cover some of the costs of production, the price the consumer had to pay for these items fell. With these lower prices came higher consumption. As demand grew, so did our production levels.

At first, subsidies might sound like a good deal for the consumer—we pay less than the cost of the item—but the truth is that they have completely distorted our eating hierarchy without actually lowering the cost of food because, after all, subsidies are just our redirected tax dollars. So what we're left with is a supermarket flooded with various iterations of the same food types.

As we produced more and more grain, our supplies eventually surpassed the demand. To help get rid of some of this overstock, we commissioned farmers and scientists to find new things to do with these surpluses. While farmers began feeding corn and wheat to animals that had never eaten these plants before—such as cows and fish—scientists ingeniously found ways to convert these crops into a variety of different forms. Some experts estimate that corn-derivative products—like high-fructose corn syrup, maltodextrin, xanthan gum, saccharin, and diglycerides—are found in nearly 90 percent of all processed foods. What we're left with are supermarket shelves lined with variations of the same few food sources, and we can see the toll it's taken on our health.

Subsidies lay the groundwork for what's currently happening in our food system. If we want to make it possible for Americans to do what's best for their health, no matter what their income is, we need to start by doing away with subsidies that make one type of food more fiscally attractive than any other.

As consumers, we can start creating the demand for affordable, accessible healthy food by making sure that we opt for organic, local, and

humanely produced items whenever possible. As the number of purchasers looking for food items like this increases, producers will make it their business to develop the amount and quality of product we demand. Moreover, it may influence our government to actually 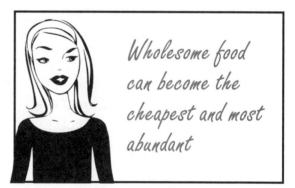 start supporting family farmers who can produce the diverse array of food we need to be healthy, so that these wholesome foods become those that are cheapest and most abundant.

Wholesome food can become the cheapest and most abundant

CONSCIOUS CHOICES

While living on campus, you have a unique opportunity to experiment with more balanced meals because most schools provide a variety of both healthy and unhealthy options for their students in the dining halls. Even if you have to pay a little, you can usually get healthy food at a very reasonable price because many meal plans are subsidized by the school. This means you have a chance to decide whether you will eat healthily or not without having cost as a primary concern. But there is always more that universities can do to be the beacon of progress for the rest of America, especially with the help of committed students like us. My hope is that if we start to place an emphasis on quality and variety, rather than solely on quantity and convenience, we might be able to send a shock wave through the system that would result in a much healthier balance for everyone, in college and beyond.

Now, I certainly don't expect you to go cold turkey (remember, nothing is off limits when you follow the Dorm Room Diet!). I know that processed, prepackaged foods are sometimes all that's available, and that you may not be fortunate enough to live in a town that has access to locally grown produce (heck, some places in this country are called "produce deserts" because you can't find fresh food anywhere!).

The aim of this chapter is just to help you understand the distinctions—what does *organic* even mean? What about *industrial agriculture*?—and figure out the places where it would be easy for you to make the "conscious choice." If we all take a few small steps in the right direction, we can nudge food industry leaders to take a look at what is currently available and invest some time, money, and energy into bringing healthier alternatives to the table. Meanwhile, we've got to start putting our money where our mouths are.

> We might send a shock wave through the system that would result in a much healthier balance for everyone

THE PLANET'S HEALTH

Eating consciously is part of the larger goal of living consciously, which means you try to take note of all the global ramifications your daily decisions may have and live as "sustainably" as possible (leaving nothing worse than the way you found it, and preferably better).

None of us lives in a vacuum: each of our actions has a *re*action, whether we notice it or not. The way that we eat affects our personal health, but it also affects our planet's health. The eating choices we make today predict the kind of food that will be available to us in the future and the way it is grown, which is why it's so important that we start looking for ways to make the most of our purchasing power today.

Ultimately, what would be best for our health and that of the planet would be if we could all eat whole, organic foods—lots of fresh fruits and veggies, depending on the season, plus whole grains and some meat, with limited additional fat and sugar and minimal processing. Ideally, these foods would be grown on local farms, so that we avoid all the mess of preservation and transportation, while supporting the industry of family farmers. With a larger number of individual farmers planting a variety of crops, we could have food offerings that changed with the seasons, and healthier soil and bodies as a result. This is because changing the crops that are planted throughout the year allows the soil to replenish lost nutrients, while providing you with access to many different nutritional resources. More organic planting would mean less hazardous exposure to unnecessary chemicals that come to us in the form of fertilizer, pesticides, and preservatives. Keeping these toxins out of our soil and our bodies would allow both to heal. Assuming this could offer us enough food to sustain our population, doesn't it sound like the obvious choice of food systems?

Of course, this is a far cry from where we are today. The industrial agriculture we have now is the product of our domestic demand for huge quantities of the same kinds of foods, available year-round at rock-bottom prices. The health problems that result from eating the same processed foods all the time (ask yourself: how many foods and beverages have you had today that included high-fructose corn syrup, sugar, or white flour as one of the first three ingredients?) are all those commonly associated with the so-called Western diet: heart disease, diabetes, cancer. These are serious diseases, all of which could likely be avoided if we just had more opportunity to choose the right foods as part of a healthy lifestyle.

As a result of our current system, it has become really difficult to be healthy in this country because the foods that are best for us are often the ones that are the most expensive and hard to find. It's all about *access*: we need healthy foods to be as available and affordable as their unhealthy alternatives so that people can at least have the *option to live healthily*.

INDUSTRIAL AGRICULTURE

Today, in America, we have something called *industrial agriculture*, and it has changed the way we eat. Fifty years ago, people had fresh milk delivered in glass bottles from a local farm, and it went bad within the week. Today, we may have pictures of pasture-grazing cattle on the milk cartons we buy at the store, but this milk can last upwards of a month, and chances are the cow it came from never saw green grass.

Industrial agriculture refers to a process of mechanizing the growing, harvesting, and processing of food. Rather than having a multitude of small family farms producing a variety of healthful, wholesome foods, we have huge, multinational, multibillion-dollar corporations that have maximized their ability to provide food by making every natural step in the life cycle of a crop or animal more "efficient" through the application of science and engineering. For instance, chickens today are raised and slaughtered (with artificially augmented breasts, since American consumers prefer white meat) in 48 days, as opposed to the 70 days it took in 1950. While this is certainly a feat of scientific achievement, the result is a much less healthy chicken—when they are engineered to grow this fast, their bones and internal organs cannot maintain the pace, and they can barely take a step or two without collapsing—and a lower-quality meat for you and me.

Similar "advancements" have been made in the way we produce beef, pork, milk, eggs, corn, soybeans, canola, and wheat. We wanted more food, produced bigger and faster, selected for the qualities we prize most, and offered to us at a fraction of what it costs to create. In the past, we gave little thought to the unintended consequences our food demands created. But it is becoming increasingly apparent that the delicate balance on which our food system operates is highly unstable; that we as consumers suffer because the overwhelming majority of foods provided by this system are not health-sustaining, yet they have reached a point where the alternatives are no longer affordable; and the longer we allow industrialized agriculture to continue, the longer it will take for us and our planet to recover.

All kind of complaints have been leveled against industrial farms and agriculture because

> *The way that we eat affects our personal health, and also our planet's health*

of the health hazards they pose, their unethical and inhumane treatment of workers and animals, and the endless amount of waste these productions create. The chemicals used to aid the growing process, the synthetic hormones and antibiotics administered to farm animals, the preservatives used to allow foods to be stored and shipped for long stretches, the contaminated water from farm runoff of animal waste, and the tons of fuel to ship the food from farm to supermarket—these are but a few of the problems with the current arrangement.

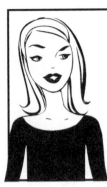

Three times a day, we have an opportunity to vote for something better

The only reason a system like this can persist is if people like us keep supporting it when we make our eating choices. Food producers will only supply what we ask for, and that is our power. Three times a day, we have an opportunity to vote for something better.

INDUSTRIAL FARMS VS. TRADITIONAL, OLD-SCHOOL FARMS

Over the last fifty years, in particular, farming has progressively been treated as a business, where efficiency is prized but quality sometimes suffers as the corporate mind-set makes profits the primary consideration. To meet the needs of a growing populace with a seemingly insatiable appetite, we instituted *industrial agriculture*, a way of mechanizing and streamlining production by making it part of one giant operation, rather than a larger number of smaller, coordinated, independent producers.

Right now, you might be asking yourself how old-school farming differs from its industrial replacement. Let's look at the growers of grains, veggies, and fruits, for instance. Old-school, family-owned farms typically grow a variety of different grain, vegetable, or fruit crops, all side by side. They've found that having this diversity acts as a natural pesticide, as different types of plants protect each other against a variety of diseases and insects. Additionally, these different kinds of plants eventually break down into the soil and act as natural fertilizers.

Through crop rotation—alternating planting one type of plant during a particular cycle or season with other types during the following cycles— farmers are able to naturally replenish the nutrients that are lost from the soil during the initial crop's growing season. As a result of this natural harmony, traditional farming does not require nearly as much synthetic fertilizer or pesticide usage, which is good for you, me, and the earth.

Industrial farms, on the other hand, typically plant only one kind of crop. They have termed this "efficient monoculture" because it allows them to easily blanket their crops with pesticides that kill everything *except* that certain plant, rather than having to work the land by hand (which would be impossible, given the farm's size). Of course, what is "efficient" for them has also increased the amount of pesticides we come into contact with in our food, elevated the toxic runoff into the water supply (rainwater washes pesticides off crops and runs downhill, or downstream, until it reaches the main body of water, where the pesticide residue collects), and with no other crops around to act as buffers, threatened the possibility that a single type of plant disease or insect could wipe out an entire farm's production.

Because they plant only one type of crop year round and season to season, industrial farms are forced to use fertilizers to replenish the stores of certain nutrients that are utterly depleted. As artificial, manmade pesticides and fertilizers build up in the soil and local water sources, they are increasingly a part of the food that eventually leaves these farms and comes to your plate.

WHAT KINDS OF FOOD SHOULD YOU CHOOSE?

When you are walking down the aisles of a supermarket, picking up a snack at the university co-op, or perusing the cafeteria options, there are a couple of identifying adjectives you want to look for when choosing what kind of food to eat. The most important things for you to know about and look for are whether the food is organic, whether it is free-range, grass-fed, and certified humane, and whether the food was grown locally.

When food is organic, free-range, grass-fed, humanely produced, and locally grown, it has likely been exposed to far fewer synthetic chemical additives, such as pesticides, fertilizers, or antibiotics. In most cases, the meat you get that is organic and grass-fed will be from healthier livestock because the animals were allowed to graze in a pasture, run around, grow naturally, and were butchered in hygienic and humane conditions. And eggs that are gathered humanely mean that they come from chickens that had open-air access and were allowed to run free and lay eggs at natural intervals. Foods that are grown nearby will also usually be fresher and more nutrient-dense because they did not have to travel many hundreds—or even thousands—of miles to get to you (a good rule of thumb is that the longer it takes get from farm to table, the fewer nutrients a particular food will have).

Industrial agriculture producers wield a tremendous amount of lobbying and advertising power (thanks to our subsidy dollars), and they are well equipped to limit how much can be said and how much can be done about their business practices. They fight hard to make it difficult for organic, free-range, humane, and local producers to advertise their food as more nutritious and safer. But you have to ask yourself: Would they really go to all the trouble of spending money to divert your attention away from their operations—to make it difficult for you, the conscious consumer, to discover what is going on, or to say anything about it if you do—if there wasn't something objectionable about them? They're worried that once you find out the truth, you might not want to buy their products anymore. And you know what? They're probably right.

IN THE NEXT FEW SECTIONS, I'll explain what organic, free-range, humane, and local mean and why they are important for your health and that of the planet. As a caveat, while these are identifiers that you should look for and try to buy as often as possible, it's way more important for you to eat as much whole, natural produce as possible. You definitely want to avoid synthetic additives—like bovine growth hormone (rBGH), genetically modified (GM) foods, and antibiotics—because these will be directly transferred from animal flesh to you, and we don't know how they will affect you long term. But if the choice is between eating conventional produce daily and organic produce once a week, I'd make sure I was getting my full servings of fruit and veggies every day and eat organic only as often as possible.

Organic

Over the past couple of years, we've been hearing more and more about organic farming. As the organic movement gains ground, it would be helpful to know a bit about what it means and why it might be better for our health than conventional growing methods.

I think the best place to start is to state precisely what the organic label means. You see it all over the place: on T-shirts and cleaning products, soap bars and pillowcases. "Organic" refers to how a raw material is grown, processed, and shipped, and tells the consumer that all of these steps maintained the original integrity of the product, so it is essentially the same as when it left the ground. Specifically this means that the product was grown without the use of toxic pesticides, synthetic fertilizers or hormones, antibiotics, genetic modification, irradiation, or sewage sludge. The U.S. Department of Agriculture (USDA) organic regulations also mandate that livestock and poultry be given "living conditions which accommodate the health and natural behavior of animals," which requires that they have to be given room to exercise, sleep, and be outdoors, at least part of the time.

NUKING FOOD

Irradiation is a process of exposing fresh produce to energy beams to kill germs and insects that cause food to spoil more quickly and could potentially lead to food poisoning. While this process keeps some produce looking nice on the shelves of our supermarkets longer, we don't know how exposure to radiation will alter the plants' chemical composition, or how our bodies will react long term to irradiated foods.

By doing without synthetic additives, organic farming contributes to keeping our water supply clean, since there is limited farm runoff of toxins. Organic farmers have developed natural ways to provide fertilizer and pest repellants by turning to biodiversity in their crops and relying on crop rotation (planting different crops at different times of the year) and composting (allowing insects and worms to turn food waste into nitrogen-rich fertilizer with tons of nutrients and minerals plants need to grow) to serve their growing needs.

The U.S. government regulates organic standards closely, so that you can have confidence in the organic label. However, because these strict guidelines are under constant attack from industrial agriculture lobbyists who want to make it more difficult for you to distinguish between their foods and organic alternatives, it takes vigilant, dedicated citizens to make sure that the standards applied to organic production methods remain strong and secure.

Critics of organic farming cite that, because this growing method is labor intensive, it cannot be relied upon to feed the world's growing population. However, a United Nations report, *Organic Agriculture and Food Security in Africa,* states that organic farming practices offer the greatest hope to developing countries because it provides jobs; boosts the income of small farmers; does not require the use of expensive seeds, chemical pesticides, or fertilizers; boosts soil quality so that it can continue to support crop growth; and can actually raise crop yields.

Here in the United States, more studies are showing that organic farming can produce yields on par with and, in some cases, superior to conventional alternatives. Research conducted by Iowa State University's Neely-Kinyon Farm has shown that the farm's organic corn, soybean, and oat crops produced as much as or more than their conventional counterparts did. Now, that's something to be excited about!

For more information on the benefits of organic farming, check out: www.organicitsworthit.org.

BUYER BEWARE

One caution: it's difficult to say how well international foods adhere to the "organic" guidelines established by the USDA, so I would stick to domestic food products labeled "organic" as much as possible.

Free-Range and Grass-fed

The term "free-range" can mean different things, depending on whether it's used to describe chickens grown for meat or for eggs. For poultry chickens, the USDA says that "free range" birds must have some access to the outdoors, though there are no specifications about what kind of environment this needs to be—it could even be a cement cage with an open ceiling. Free-range actually means nothing (yet) for egg-laying hens, so they don't necessarily get any outdoor access at all.

When it comes to grass-fed, the best possible situation is for the animal to have been allowed to graze in pasture. This gives them access to all different varieties of vegetation, and guarantees that they spent some time exercising and being in fresh air. Grass-fed, in particular, does not require that animals be raised on a pasture, but it's a good clue that producers are thinking about the health of their animals and are supplementing their diet with at least some grass. Of course, if the label says "pasture-fed," that's even better!

Certified Humane

Humane is yet another protection against those producers who try to use only minimally improved living conditions for livestock, such as "free-range," "grass-fed," and the like. For something to be considered "certified humane," it must be shown that the animals lived essentially as they would on any regular farm, without any alteration to their natural life cycle. They must be given open space in which to wander and graze, no claustrophobic confinement in tiny cages or crates, and shelter from the elements. They are not treated with any artificial growth hormones or antibiotics, and must be butchered as quickly and painlessly as possible to limit stress. In the case of eggs, certified humane products are harvested from free-nesting hens. Certified humane is the gold standard of product labeling if you're looking for wholesome, naturally produced food.

Local

Locally produced food is probably the easiest to explain because there's no fudging of the facts. Whereas guidelines for what qualifies as organic, free-range, grass-fed, or humane can sometimes vary, you should be able to find out where something is produced. If the farm a food comes from is more than 100 miles from where you're eating it, it usually isn't considered local. Still, eating foods from a few hundred miles away is better than eating foods from a few thousand miles away. Moreover, the strict regulations the USDA and Food and Drug Administration (FDA) place on how foods can be produced and treated within the United States do not apply to foods that are imported for consumption in the United States. For instance, many of our grapes come from Mexico and Chile. For farmers in each of these countries, it is not illegal to use human refuse and feces as fertilizer to grow crops. Pretty gross, huh?

And remember, the longer a food has to travel to reach you, the more likely it has been treated with preservatives or by irradiation. Along the way, these foods lose many of their natural, essential nutrients. Eating local foods supports the family farms in your area, but it also ensures that you are getting the most nutritional value for your money.

BECOME A LOCAVORE

In some cases, it is also cheaper to buy local because you cut out all the transportation and storage costs. So get out to a local farmer's market, set up home or dorm delivery of weekly produce from a local farm, join a co-op, or establish a farm-to-school program. Even better, see if you can pay a visit to a local farm and help plant or harvest! Being a part of the process takes you that much closer to the source of your food—once you taste a fresh fruit or veggie you picked off the vine, you'll be hooked.

CONSUMER ENTITLEMENT

So what's the take-away message here? Well, first and foremost, I hope you now feel equipped to make educated eating choices when it comes to selecting foods that promote your health and that of the planet. I also hope you've seen what a huge role you have to play in making sure that our food supply gets better, not worse. We ultimately provide the demand that food producers will seek to supply, so as we purchase more and more of the organic, free-range, grass-fed, certified humane, local foods, we will begin to shift the market toward quality. Industrial farmers will change their practices to meet our needs, but we need to create the demand first by reevaluating our eating values.

We have allowed a culture of "entitled consumerism" to develop, in which we feel deserving of as much food as we can possibly eat, at minimal cost, available year round and the world over. We have focused all of our attention on making sure that these demands are met, even as it becomes clear that the sad state of our populace's health is directly related to our inability to eat in sync with our nutritional needs. Correspondingly, we've paid progressively less and less attention to where our food comes from or how it is produced—whether it's strawberries in the dead of winter, or the traditional Fourth of July hot dog—and this has allowed our food system to deteriorate to the point where it is now.

When it comes to the state of our food, we have to look out for ourselves. Even as industrial agriculture giants use their profits to fund massive advertising campaigns promoting their products, their lobbyists work hard in Washington to keep any legislation from being passed that would hinder their business operations. Even more debilitating is the fact that there is a revolving door between the people in charge at our regulatory agencies—the Food and Drug Administration and the U.S. Department of Agriculture—and the executives of the very companies and groups these agencies are meant to be policing.

The conflict of interest is obvious, and the outcome is less and less oversight for the growing number of violations of human-, animal-, and environmental-health codes within industrial agriculture. Consumer rights and food safety activists have had to fight tooth and nail for the limited product labeling that is required today against agribusinesses, which do not want to be compelled by law to tell us where and how our food is produced. The less we know, the less able we are to fight for our own right to health.

Though it may seem that industry is better protected than the consumers in this regard, we have power in numbers. Fortunately, you now have a solid base of information from which to start making conscious-eating decisions that support sustainable agriculture. Every food dollar you spend is an opportunity to start to swing the pendulum back in our favor.

A FORCE FOR CHANGE

You can start by getting your college or university administration to spend their cafeteria money wisely by organizing farm-to-school programs that supply campuses with local produce. Colleges spend more than $4 billion annually on food, and this purchasing power, combined with their educational missions and community impact, means that campuses can be a hotbed of innovation and a leader in the move toward a healthier America. So many important social changes—women's suffrage, civil rights, peace movements—have been catalyzed by a few passionate young people who started the wave of enlightened national consciousness. Now, it's our turn. If we speak up forcefully, we can help create a food supply that is overwhelmed by healthy, high-quality, nutrient-filled food that is affordable for everyone. Wouldn't that be a nice legacy?

ACTION PLAN

It is important to become involved in what food is available so that you have the essential access to make healthful decisions every day. I grew up purely vegetarian, and though I did reincorporate a small amount of meat into my diet, it was crucial for me to find ways to have protein without resorting to the "mystery meat" served at the cafeteria. In high school, I managed to work closely with cafeteria staff and the school administration to implement a whole slew of new health initiatives, including student-submitted vegetarian recipes, daily salad and soup bar options, and Odwalla juice to replace soda on campus. This kind of change could take place on a much larger scale on college campuses if universities harnessed their purchasing power and their role as educators to blaze a trail toward health stewardship in America. As concerned students, we just have to push them in the right direction. For those not looking to go head-to-head with the university president, here are a couple of smaller-scale options:

Consult your cafeteria staff. Often there are things in the fridge that the cafeteria workers do not make available because they may be unaware that anyone wants them. Make a point of telling the head chef or purchaser for your cafeteria about any of your allergies or specific food needs, and more often than not, they will find a way to accommodate your needs.

See whether you can establish a farm-to-school program. This is a trend that is sweeping the nation, as more and more schools invest in purchasing a portion or a majority of their cafeteria supplies from local producers. It saves on transportation costs, and the result is fresher, more wholesome food for everyone!

Food shop, too. Once a week, I borrowed a friend's car and ran to the local grocery store near my college. We were fortunate to have an independent health food store very near campus, and I would buy my main foodstuffs and snacks there, supplementing with salad items, whole grains, and cereals from the cafeteria.

Start a farmer's market. While I was in college, one of my best friends established the first farmer's market run fully by students. It came to campus every Tuesday and flooded the commons with fruits and vegetables, local dairy products, fresh bakery bread, and a slew of other delicious goodies. Depending on where you live, the local farmers and food producers are generally thrilled to partner with the surrounding community, both to gain exposure and to sell their products directly.

STEP 10

GET COOKING

Recipes You Can Enjoy

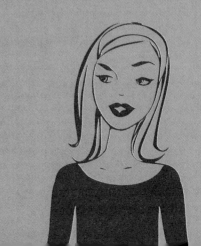

COOKING FOR YOURSELF is a great way to get conscious about where your food comes from and to know how it is prepared. Plus, it gives you an alternative to the processed junk food too often available on college campuses. In this chapter, you'll be amazed at how easy it is to make some of your own meals and snacks, even if it's only a couple of times a week.

Part of the thrill—and the stress—of moving away from home is the idea that from now on you will be responsible for all of your meals. Whether you're eating at the cafeteria, in the dorm, or out at a restaurant, the decision about what you eat is all yours. Even when you make some occasional visits home, you might find that you're given a lot more freedom about what you choose to eat—especially if you bring an array of quick-and-healthy recipes home with you.

In this chapter, we'll explore some of my favorite recipes for breakfast, lunch, and dinner (and some of my friends' college specialties, too), as well as a few convenient snacks that helped me beat those midafternoon junk-food cravings. I love to cook, but I especially love cooking on the fly, where you don't need a ton of fancy equipment or ingredients. Food that tastes good, and is good for you, doesn't need to take a lot of time or even skill (though it helps if you know what you like). In fact, most of the recipes you'll find here only require a measuring cup, a mixing bowl, and your hands!

I picked some especially simple recipes for this chapter, since I know how difficult it can be to find time and space to cook while you're at school. You'll find a range of flavors and some interesting takes on old favorites. Before we get started, I want to tell you a bit about how this chapter is structured.

The recipes have been arranged in four sections: breakfast, lunch, dinner, and snacks. I've designated three levels of difficulty (one, two, and three carrots) for the recipes, depending on the kind of equipment you'll need to make them. With any equipment, you should read the owner's manual to make sure you operate it properly.

Level 1 (one carrot): These recipes are made by hand, without any equipment. All you'll need in most cases is a mixing bowl, a spoon, and a measuring cup.

Level 2 (two carrots): These recipes require either a rice cooker or a blender. The rice cooker serves many purposes—from perfectly cooking rice and beans to being the ideal soup pot—and is a breeze to use (mine literally has one button). Other recipes call for a blender, which is a great thing to have on hand for smoothies and shakes, as well as puréed soups. Most blenders have a variety of mixing and blending options, which just means more opportunity for experimenting! The recipes in this chapter will tell you which option to select, so don't worry about having to guess.

Level 3 🥕🥕🥕 (three carrots):   If your dorm has a kitchen-ette with a stove, a microwave, and/or an oven, or if you live in a house or apartment, level three recipes give you something a little more complex to try (and you can also test these out on your family the next time you're home).

Keep in mind that these are just a few of my favorite recipes, and they're meant to inspire you to experiment on your own. Once you get comfortable in the kitchen, you can (and should!) start experimenting with new recipes that allow you to taste different flavors and enjoy different kinds of food. Having variety in your diet helps to ensure that you're get-ting balanced nutrition, keeps your taste buds from getting bored, and makes sure your healthy lifestyle is one that's full of zest!

The following recipes are portioned for one person, unless otherwise in-dicated.

Here are some basic guidelines to keep in mind when preparing the recipes:

1. As we discussed in the last chapter, as many ingredients as possible should be organic, whenever you have the option. Still, it's better to eat fresh vegetables and fruits (or even canned and frozen varieties) as often as possible, rather than waiting for the organic version to become available. Just make sure you wash fresh conventional produce with a good produce cleaning spray or rinse just a minute under running warm water if you don't have spray. Washing with a produce spray helps get rid of a lot of the toxic chemicals used to preserve food during shipping, which you definitely don't want to end up in your finished products.

2. High-fructose corn syrup and hydrogenated fats should be avoided at all costs. Even though the FDA has sanctioned these ingredients, we don't really know what their long-term health effects are, and some studies have linked them to weight gain due to overeating, possibly because they mess with your body's ability to tell when you're full.

3. Choose sweetened-with-sugar items rather than ones with artificial sweeteners—the couple of extra calories are preferable to all the chemicals, as long as you eat them in moderation.

4. Low-fat dairy is a fine choice, provided that all the fat isn't replaced by added sodium, sugar, or artificial sweeteners.

5. Whenever possible, choose sea salt and fresh-cracked pepper— you'll find the flavor is much more intense (the same is true of fresh herbs, though dried herbs are totally fine in a pinch).

BREAKFAST

At breakfast, there are a few specific goals you should aim for. First of all, you want to let your body (and your metabolism) know you are awake, so that it revs back up after a night of sleep. You want to make sure you get some protein and complex carbohydrates for fuel, and little bit of healthy fat is good to make sure you stay full. Fiber is also something that's great with every meal, but it's especially good at breakfast because it helps regulate your blood sugar and that helps curb your appetite throughout the day. Even if you only have five minutes, whip up one of the following easy breakfast solutions to start your day off right!

A BIG BREAKFAST

I always try to live by the adage: breakfast like a king, lunch like a prince, and dine like a pauper. In other words, have your biggest meal earlier in the day to make sure you have time to use the calories.

---

1. *Nuttier Butter*

½ cup peanut butter
½ cup almond butter
½ cup cashew or hazelnut butter
1 cup flax seeds

YIELD: 2½ cups SERVING SIZE: 1 tbsp

CALORIES: 50 TOTAL FAT: 4.3 g FIBER: 1.4 g PROTEIN: 1.8 g

Mix all ingredients together for a powerful protein snack, loaded with good-for-you omega fats.

Eat a teaspoon on its own for an energy jolt, or try spreading some on celery sticks or rice cakes.

2. *Banana Nut Oatmeal*

1 cup water
½ cup original oats
1 ripe banana, sliced
1 tsp coconut oil
6 walnuts (optional)

YIELD: ½ cup

CALORIES: 464 TOTAL FAT: 14.3 g FIBER: 11 g PROTEIN: 15 g

Bring water to a boil and add oats. Reduce heat and stir occasionally, until water is ¾ evaporated. Add sliced banana, continuing to stir until all water is evaporated. Melt in coconut oil and add walnuts, chopped, if so desired.

This has tons of protein, some good omega fats from the coconut oil, and a great dose of complex carbs and fiber that will keep you full all morning. (Research shows that people who start the day with oatmeal stabilize their blood sugar and are better able to maintain a healthy weight!)

3. Breakfast Sandwich (sweet)

1 slice whole grain or millet bread (gluten-free)
1 tsp nuttier butter (see page 257 for recipe)
1 banana

CALORIES: 190.6 TOTAL FAT: 2.9 g FIBER: 5.5 g PROTEIN: 5.4 g

Toast the bread. If you prefer, you can cut it in half, creating two thinner pieces of toast and giving your sandwich a top and a bottom. I love open-faced sandwiches because I think it allows the flavors to come out better. Spread the nuttier butter mixture on the toast, and top with sliced banana.

My grandpa would always put honey and raisins on top (he called it a "Gypsy Sandwich"), but that adds a bunch of sugar, so I would stick with the basics, which pack a ton of protein and potassium, and lots of healthy fiber to keep your digestive tract moving smoothly.

4. *Breakfast Sandwich (savory)* 🥕🥕🥕🥕

  1 slice whole grain or millet bread (gluten-free)

  1 scrambled egg, or 2 scrambled egg whites

  1 tsp coconut oil

  ¼ cup refried beans or cooked black beans (or mashed sweet
    potato)

  ¼ cup salsa of your choice

  Tabasco, to your desired spiciness

  CALORIES: 210 TOTAL FAT: 9 g FIBER: 4.7 g PROTEIN: 12.1 g

Toast the bread. If you prefer, you can cut it in half, creating two thinner pieces of toast and giving your sandwich a top and bottom. Scramble the eggs, using coconut oil to grease the pan if needed. Spread the bread with your refried bean mixture (you could also use mashed sweet potato, for a sweeter variation). Put the scrambled eggs on top of this layer, and top off with salsa and a dash of Tabasco for added spice.

You'll be getting lots of protein, plus the cayenne in Tabasco is a natural appetite suppressant, and the salsa gives a nice flavor boost without many calories or any fat.

5. *Greek Yogurt with Honey and Chopped Walnuts* 🥕

  ½ cup strained Greek yogurt, low-fat or fat-free

  1 tbsp honey, drizzled over top

  8 walnuts, chopped

Add the walnuts as a topping on the yogurt and drizzle with honey.

  YIELD: ½ cup

  CALORIES: 308 TOTAL FAT: 18.3 g FIBER: 1.9 g PROTEIN: 12.7 g

259

A Mediterranean specialty that is perfect for a quick breakfast or post-workout snack, this dish is super easy to make and always good to have on hand. The yogurt is laden with protein and calcium, while the walnuts add some healthy omega fats to keep you energized and feeling full longer.

WALNUTS TURKISH STYLE

My family loves walnuts—we eat them the traditional Turkish way by soaking them in water overnight. This simple step takes away any of the bitterness, and actually helps your body absorb the important vitamins and nutrients walnuts have to offer by neutralizing the enzyme inhibitors in each nut. Walnuts are loaded with omega-3 fatty acids (the good fats that keep your hair, nails, and skin looking hydrated and healthy), and have tons of fiber, too, so they're a great snack on the run that will help you feel full longer.

---

6. *Breakfast Parfait*

1 cup yogurt, cow or goat, plain or low-fat flavor (always make sure you choose varieties that are naturally low in sugar—stay away from high-fructose corn syrup, though)

½ cup mixed berries, blended frozen or fresh

½ cup low-sugar granola (again, no artificial sweeteners, please!) (or, if you prefer, crushed walnuts or almonds)

YIELD: 2 cups

CALORIES: 338 TOTAL FAT: 6.2 g FIBER: 4 g PROTEIN: 15.8 g

Alternate a dollop of yogurt with a sprinkling of berries and then granola (or crushed nuts) in a cup until you've reached your desired portion. These cups can be prepared a day or two in advance so you can take one with you on the run!

7. *Banana Almond Smoothie*

½ cup plain or vanilla yogurt, sweetened with sugar

1 ripe banana, sliced

1 tbsp almond butter

1 tbsp psyllium husk

1 scoop vanilla whey protein powder (optional)

¼ cup almond milk, or regular low-fat or fat-free milk

1 cup ice

Add honey if needed for extra sweetness

YIELD: 2 cups

CALORIES: 340 (430 with protein powder) TOTAL FAT: 11.4 g
FIBER: 7.7 g PROTEIN: 15 g (31.4 g with protein powder)

Whir in a blender until smooth and creamy. This is a sumptuously sweet, decadently nutty smoothie for those mornings when you're craving a heartier breakfast.

You can add the protein powder if you feel like you could use it— maybe you've had a couple of hard workouts this week—or skip it, since the yogurt also provides some protein, plus natural probiotic bacteria that helps maintain optimal health in your digestive tract. Psyllium husks offer tons of soluble fiber, which help clean your digestive tract as well. You're also going to get protein and omega fats from the almond butter, and potassium from the banana. A delicious, nutrient-packed delight!

8. *Superfood Breakfast Smoothie*

½ cup yogurt, plain or sweetened with sugar

1 cup fresh fruit of your choosing, plus at least ½ banana

1 tsp honey, if needed

1 tbsp psyllium husks

1 cup ice (or use frozen fruit and skip ice)

YIELD: 2½ cups

CALORIES: 435 TOTAL FAT: 4.5 g FIBER: 11.8 g PROTEIN: 8.8 g

Optional: Add the contents of 2 Ester-C capsules along with a capful of an algae or chlorophyll supplement (any health food store will have one) and one serving bee pollen for an extra energy boost and an easy way to get some of your vitamins.

Whir all ingredients in a blender until smooth and creamy.

Psyllium husks help clean your digestive tract and expand with water, so that you'll be nice and full. And if you add the optional vitamin supplements, it packs a powerful vitamin punch. Enjoy!

LUNCH

At lunch, you're usually looking for something a bit more savory than sweet, and you probably won't have a ton of time to whip up something like chili when you're darting between classes. Again, some of the things to look for in your lunch foods are fiber, complex carbohydrates and protein, and, of course, a big healthy serving or two of veggies, with fruit for dessert. Sandwiches on whole wheat bread with a healthy side salad are a great combo. A big salad with sliced turkey or tofu or kidney beans is also a great option. Keep this meal a little smaller than breakfast, unless you have a big sporting event or a workout class coming up in the afternoon where you'll need some additional energy and fuel to function your best.

9. Miso Soup

¼ cup dried wakame (Japanese seaweed, if desired)
¼ cup chopped tofu, firm (if desired)
1 cup hot water (not boiling—boiling water kills the good enzymes in miso)
1 tbsp miso paste

YIELD: 1 cup

CALORIES: 63 TOTAL FAT: 2.1 g FIBER: 0 g PROTEIN: 5.1 g

Mix the wakame and tofu into hot water, and then add the miso paste last, and voilà! I love to make this ahead of time and it keeps well in the fridge for three days, so you can warm it up for soup on the go. It's a delicious snack or part of a meal that is loaded with nutrients, enzymes, and minerals (seaweed is nature's superfood).

10. Kale Chips

1 head of kale
¼ cup olive oil
2 tbsp salt, sea salt preferred
Seasonings to taste (optional)

YIELD: 6 servings PER SERVING: CALORIES: 64

TOTAL FAT: 5.8 g FIBER: .16 g PROTEIN: .3 g

Cut off bite-sized pieces of kale after washing and drying thoroughly. Using your fingertips, brush all pieces front and back with some olive oil, and lay in a single layer on a cookie sheet. Sprinkle with salt and any other seasonings you like (I sometimes use garlic salt, or add flavorings like cumin or curry for some added zest). Bake for 8 minutes at 315 degrees—crunchy goodness!

11. Kale Salad

1 head of kale
¼ cup olive oil
1 tsp salt
1 lemon, juiced
Salt and pepper to taste
¼ cup hemp seeds

YIELD: 6 servings PER SERVING: CALORIES: 190

TOTAL FAT: 6.6 g FIBER: 5.3 g PROTEIN: 9.3 g

Thoroughly wash and dry kale. Tear into bite-sized pieces and place in salad bowl. Pour olive oil and salt on top, and using your fingertips, massage the kale until it begins to soften. Sprinkle lemon juice to taste, and more salt and pepper, if needed. Add hemp seeds for added protein and good omega fats, and you're ready to go.

12. Gazpacho

1 diced tomato
¼ cup diced onion
½ diced jalapeño (Be sure to wear gloves when you're cutting, or wash your hands thoroughly! Don't want any jalapeño getting in your eye—it stings!)
1 diced cucumber

Salt and pepper to taste
Optional: ½ tsp sour cream and cucumber

YIELD: 1 cup

CALORIES: 38.6 TOTAL FAT: .5 g FIBER: 2.2 g PROTEIN: 2.2 g

Blend all ingredients on high in your blender (give it a rest from the margaritas) until you reach the desired consistency. I like mine a little bit chunky, more like a salsa than tomato soup. You can add ½ tsp sour cream if you like, though I think it's perfect alone. I also add a couple of cucumber slices on the plate to eat alongside for extra crunch and fiber.

13. Crunchy Avocado Salad

1 ripe avocado
½ cup sliced cucumber, Persian or English
½ cup cherry tomatoes, grape tomatoes, or chopped tomatoes
Juice from ½ lime
Sea salt to taste

CALORIES: 418 TOTAL FAT: 35.8 g FIBER: 17.4 g PROTEIN: 6 g

This is basically an über-chunky guacamole. Chop avocado into ¾-inch cubes and place in a bowl. Add cucumber and tomatoes and lime. Stir gently and salt to taste.

The avocado is calorie-dense, but these calories come from the great omega fats that avocados are so rich in. Also, cucumbers have tons of water and fiber, which will help to keep you full and hydrated. Especially in the summer months, when all these fruits and veggies are readily available, this is a nutrient-dense and satisfyingly crunchy new spin on salad. Serve with kale chips or toasted, whole wheat pita chips.

Recipe courtesy of Laura Trice, MD, author of The Wholesome Junk Food Cookbook: More than 100 Healthy Recipes for Everyday Snacking. *Used by kind permission of Running Press, copyright 2009.*

14. Vegan Tofu Dog Sandwich

1 tofu dog (vegetarian hot dog substitute)
1 slice whole wheat, whole grain, or millet (gluten-free) bread
Vegenaise (mayo substitute, tastes amazing!)
Yellow mustard
Ketchup (non–high-fructose corn syrup!)

CALORIES: 281 TOTAL FAT: 12.7 g FIBER: 3 g PROTEIN: 12.3 g

Put the tofu dog, which comes frozen, in a bowl with just enough water to cover it in the microwave for 1 minute. Test if the dog is hot. If not, another minute in the microwave is needed. The tofu dog should be hot in the center before eating. Toast the bread and slice in half lengthwise, so you get two equally sized, thinner slices. Spread a thin layer of Vegenaise on one or both halves. Slice the tofu dog lengthwise, and lay across bread. Spread as much mustard as you'd like and 1 tablespoon ketchup on the other half of the bread (or you can squirt ketchup and mustard over the hot dog itself).

This sandwich is so easy to make, cruelty-free, and packs a ton of fiber and vegetarian protein!

15. Lentil Salad

1 cup lentils

2 cups water

1 bunch chives, chopped

1 clove garlic, pressed

2 tbsp olive oil

2 tbsp red wine vinegar

Salt and pepper to taste

Optional: Diced red pepper, celery, and carrots

YIELD: Two servings PER SERVING: CALORIES: 254

TOTAL FAT: 14.3 g FIBER: 9.1 g PROTEIN: 10.7 g

Boil the lentils and water in your rice cooker, until water is boiled off and lentils are tender but not mushy. Add remaining ingredients, making sure to add ½ of each recommended amount and then taste so you get a lentil salad you will love!

You can add diced red pepper to this for some nice color and nutrients, or even diced celery and carrots to sneak some more vegetables in. I'm a fan of a very simple lentil salad over mixed greens, with a simple vinaigrette (see next recipe) on top. This should make enough for two or three portions, so be sure to have Tupperware containers on hand to save for tomorrow or the next day!

16. Simple Vinaigrette (sweet)

2 tbsp olive oil

2 tbsp balsamic vinegar

½ tsp mustard, yellow or Dijon

½ tsp soy sauce

½ tsp honey

Salt and pepper to taste

YIELD: 6 servings **PER SERVING: CALORIES:** 52.3

TOTAL FAT: 4.5 g **FIBER:** .03 g **PROTEIN:** .1 g

Mix well.

17. Simple Vinaigrette (savory)

2 tbsp olive oil
2 tbsp white-wine vinegar
½ tsp mustard, yellow or Dijon
Salt and pepper to taste

YIELD: 4 servings **PER SERVING: CALORIES:** 62

TOTAL FAT: 6.8 g **FIBER:** .05 g **PROTEIN:** .05 g

Mix well.

18. Citrus Vinaigrette (sweet)

2 tbsp olive oil
2 tbsp red-wine vinegar
1 tbsp orange juice
Salt and pepper to taste

YIELD: 4 servings **PER SERVING: CALORIES:** 62.5

TOTAL FAT: 6.8 g **FIBER:** 0 g **PROTEIN:** .03 g

Mix well.

19. Garlic Greens

1/3 cup onions, diced

2 cloves garlic, pressed

2 tbsp olive oil

1 head spinach, kale, bok choy, broccoli rabe, collard greens
   (basically, anything you have on hand)

3 tbsp water

Salt and pepper to taste

YIELD: 1½ cups

CALORIES: 337 TOTAL FAT: 28 g FIBER: 8 g PROTEIN: 9 g

Place onions, garlic, and oil in a medium-heat skillet/saucepan and sauté until onions turn translucent. Add all remaining ingredients and cover. As the greens start to wilt and condense, uncover to get a crispier green (more water can evaporate without the lid on, but you need it on originally to let the greens steam a bit). If you don't want them crispy, leave the lid on until they start to wilt, then take the lid off and sauté in the garlic and oil for only about a minute more before enjoying.

20. Spinach Soup

½ cup water, plus 2 cups (you can substitute vegetable broth, if
   you like, or add a bouillon cube to the water)

1 clove garlic, pressed

1 bunch spinach

Barley, brown rice, or lentils (optional)

YIELD: 2 servings

CALORIES: 87 TOTAL FAT: 1 g FIBER: 3.2 g PROTEIN: 4.3 g

Add 2 cups of hot water or broth (or add bouillon cube to water to make broth) to the garlic and spinach. Purée in blender or leave liquid and add barley, brown rice, or lentils, if desired.

DINNER

At dinner, you want to try to keep your meal as light as possible. Lean proteins and lots of veggies are always a good option. So are hearty soups and salads. Another great choice is just to eat half the portion you might eat at lunch—so half a veggie burger, or half a portion of grains or legumes, like quinoa and lentils, paired with lots of leafy greens. At dinner, you'll probably have a bit more time to prepare your meal, so make sure that whatever you decide to eat, it's something that helps you relax and refuel after a long day. You could even think about preparing some leftovers for breakfast or lunch the next day!

21. Brown Rice with Vegetables

½ cup brown rice

2 cups water

1 tsp olive oil or coconut oil

½ tsp salt

1 clove garlic, pressed

¼ cup chopped onion

½ cup chopped carrot

½ cup chopped celery

(You can add broccoli, kale, whatever you have on hand. It
  will take some experimenting to know how much water is
  required.)

YIELD: 2 servings PER SERVING: CALORIES: 149

TOTAL FAT: 7.4 g FIBER: 4.5 g PROTEIN: 3.3 g

Put all these ingredients in the rice cooker and let them do their thing! When all the water is boiled off, your rice and vegetables should be tender and full of flavor. (For more flavor, add an all-natural bouillon cube to the water before turning the rice cooker on.)

Brown rice is an excellent complex carbohydrate, loaded with fiber and healthy energy sugars. By making it in the rice cooker all at once, you spare yourself having to prepare the vegetables separately: they will be perfectly steamed and blended with the rice—ready to eat!

22. Three Bean Vegetarian Chili

1 can tomato sauce
½ can each, kidney beans, black beans, pinto beans, precooked
½ cup vegetarian meat, either slices of tofu dogs or vegetarian crumbled beef substitute (optional)
½ cup brown rice with vegetables (see recipe above)

YIELD: 3 servings PER SERVING: CALORIES: 126

TOTAL FAT: 1.6 g FIBER: 10.7 g PROTEIN: 14.4 g

Because the tomato sauce is already seasoned, you barely have to lift a finger to prepare this delicious dish. Combine the tomato sauce and precooked beans in a pot and bring to a boil. Once boiling, reduce heat to a simmer and cover to allow all the flavors to meld together. Ladle over vegetarian meat and brown rice for an incredibly filling, supremely easy, fiber- and protein-packed meal.

23. Brussels Sprout Chips

1 lb Brussels sprouts (or, enough to fill up a large cooking bowl)
½ cup olive oil

Salt and pepper to taste

YIELD: 4 servings PER SERVING: CALORIES: 270

TOTAL FAT: 25 g FIBER: 4.3 g PROTEIN: 3.8 g

Preheat your oven/toaster oven to 400 degrees. Cut the ends off the sprouts. Peel as many leaves as will come off easily, and toss them into a large bowl. After peeling, cut the hearts into 4 pieces, and toss those in the bowl, too. With an oil spritzer, spray just enough olive oil to lightly coat the pieces, mixing well (use as much olive oil as it takes to evenly but lightly coat all the pieces). Sprinkle salt and pepper to taste (less is more with the salt; you can always add more after baking), and mix well.

On a large baking sheet lined with parchment paper, spread the Brussels sprouts into one even layer. Put them in the oven. In about 10 minutes, check the sprouts. Some leaves brown faster than others, so remove any crisp, brown leaves from the sheet, and place them in a serving bowl. Turn the rest with a large spoon, and return to the oven. Check again in about 5 minutes.

At this point, most of the individual leaves should be ready, leaving only the hearts on the baking sheet. Flip the hearts, and leave in the oven for 5 more minutes. Once the hearts are tender and browned, add them to the serving bowl with the rest of the leaves.

Now, stand back and watch your family/guests pig out on vegetables.

(Courtesy Haley Pierson-Cox—http://thezenofmaking.blogspot.com)

24. Quinoa with Veggies

½ cup water
½ cup quinoa

¼ cup frozen spinach, thawed and squeezed dry of liquid

½ can low-sodium garbanzo beans, rinsed

½ package beluga lentils

1 roma tomato, chopped

1 pinch of salt

1 pinch of garlic powder

Dash of paprika

$^1/_8$ cup low-moisture vegetable rennet mozzarella cheese, shredded (optional)

YIELD: 2 cups

CALORIES: 483 TOTAL FAT: 10.2 g FIBER: 19.8 g PROTEIN: 31.3 g

Place the water in a microwave-safe bowl, and microwave for 3 minutes or until boiling. Once boiled, add quinoa and cover with a plate so that the quinoa rises. Place the spinach, garbanzo beans, lentils, and tomato together in the bowl with the quinoa. Add a pinch of salt, garlic powder, and a dash of paprika. Finish with low-moisture shredded cheese, if desired.

This is a great, hearty dish that serves as a nice substitute for pasta. Quinoa is gluten-free and loaded with protein—the Aztecs actually harvested it for their long journeys through the mountains because it was so densely packed with nutrients. You might not be preparing for a three-day trek, but quinoa is one way to make sure you never run out of fuel, and it's quick and easy, too!

(Courtesy Alexandra Kirsch)

25. Tofu Stir-fry with Asparagus and Green Beans

1 tbsp extra virgin olive oil

3 cloves garlic, minced

1 package of extra firm tofu, cubed

1 lb asparagus, cleaned

1 lb green beans, cleaned

2 tbsp low-sodium soy sauce

2 tbsp dried ginger

1 green onion, chopped

Handful of bean sprouts

YIELD: 4 servings **PER SERVING: CALORIES:** 115

TOTAL FAT: 4.3 g **FIBER:** 6.4 g **PROTEIN:** 6.9 g

Heat oil with garlic on stove over medium heat. Place tofu in pan with the asparagus and the green beans. Cook for 10 minutes, stirring frequently. Add soy sauce, ginger, onion, and garlic powder. Place heat on low, cover pan, stirring every minute or so, until soy sauce combines with ginger to make a slightly thick sauce. Garnish with more green onion and bean sprouts. This recipe gets in a ton of your daily vegetables, and a good vegetable protein source in the tofu, while adding a little Asian flair to your weekly menu.

(Courtesy Alexandra Kirsch)

26. *Roasted Vegetables*

1 medium sweet potato, sliced

1 red pepper, julienned

1 red onion, sliced

1 can low-sodium garbanzo beans, rinsed

1 lb asparagus, cut in half

2 tbsp extra virgin olive oil

1 pinch of salt

1 pinch of garlic powder

1 pinch of dried basil

1 pinch of paprika

1 pinch of pepper

YIELD: 3 servings PER SERVING: CALORIES: 328

TOTAL FAT: 15 g FIBER: 10.3 g PROTEIN: 9.1 g

Preheat oven to 400 degrees. Place vegetables on a cookie sheet, pouring the olive oil over them, using hands to make sure oil is evenly spread. Add spices and rub with hands over all vegetables. Cook at 400 degrees for 40 minutes.

So easy to make and these also keep really well! They're great as a side dish or meal the night you make them, and the next day I like to layer a selection of roasted veggies over a piece of whole grain toast spread with hummus for a hearty and flavorful sandwich, loaded with nutrients, protein, and complex carbohydrates.

(Courtesy Alexandra Kirsch)

27. *Black Bean, Chickpea, Lentil Burgers*

1 can low-sodium black beans, rinsed

1 can low-sodium chickpeas, rinsed

1 package packaged beluga lentils

1 egg

1½ tbsp flour

Nonfat cooking spray

Garlic powder to taste

Pepper to taste

YIELD: 3 servings PER SERVING: CALORIES: 210

TOTAL FAT: 1.6 g FIBER: 8.6 g PROTEIN: 12.7 g

Preheat oven to 375 degrees. Using a blender, blend ingredients (except the cooking spray) until coarse. If the mixture is too thin, it will not cook properly in the oven. Spray nonfat cooking spray on your hands to prevent the mixture from sticking. Make equal-size patties and place them on a foil-covered cookie sheet. Spray a small amount of cooking spray on each patty to make sure they brown on top and do not burn.

Serve with salsa, or a little yogurt mixed with 1 tbsp olive oil and garlic salt to taste. These are a great alternative to regular burgers, whether you're at a tailgate party or grilling for your family. Crammed with protein and flavor, too, these just might turn some nonbelievers on to vegetarianism!

(Courtesy Alexandra Kirsch)

28. Candied Sweet Potato

1 small sweet potato
1 tsp coconut oil
Agave, if you want it sweeter ("candied")

CALORIES: 153 TOTAL FAT: 4.7 g FIBER: 4.7 g PROTEIN: 2.4 g

Stab a small sweet potato 8 times all over with a fork (if you don't, it will explode), and put it in the microwave on high for ten minutes (or in an oven at 400 degrees for 10 minutes). Rotate and replace it in the microwave oven for 5 more minutes (time will vary depending on the size of the potato). You should be able to make a permanent indent by pushing your finger against the skin. Cut the potato open to make sure it is cooked through (all flesh should be tender, not hard). Add the coconut oil and allow it to melt, and then mix, either in the skin or you can remove all the orange insides and mix in a bowl. Add 1 teaspoon agave if you want it sweeter.

SNACKS

If you don't have anything that feels like a special treat, what fun is that!

29. Stuffed Dates (vegan, raw, no appliances needed)

2 dates or dried figs
2 walnut halves
1 tsp coconut oil, softened
½ cup shredded, unsweetened coconut

CALORIES: 854 TOTAL FAT: 71.3 g FIBER: 19.7 g PROTEIN: 8.3 g

Cut a small slit in each date and take out the pit, replacing it with a walnut half. Using your finger, coat the outside of the date with softened coconut oil, and roll in the shredded coconut.

There's not a ton of nutritional benefit to this recipe—it's just delicious and it reminds me of my Turkish grandparents, who always have a plate of dried fruit and nuts on the table for dessert when I go to visit them. Still, walnuts are thought to help with eyesight, and have some good omega fats! Remember: you want to keep all nuts in the refrigerator until you use them because their oils can go rancid if left out at room temperature for too long.

My good friend, Dr. Laura Trice of Laura's Wholesome Junk Food was kind enough to share the inspiration for this recipe with us. Her cookbook is a great resource for healthfully satisfying a sweet-tooth!

Recipe from The Wholesome Junk Food Cookbook: More than 100 Healthy Recipes for Everyday Snacking, *by Laura Trice, MD. Used by kind permission from Running Press, copyright 2009.*

30. *Fruit Compote*

1 cup mixed berries, frozen
1 tsp sugar
1 lemon, juiced

CALORIES: 95 TOTAL FAT: 0.3 g FIBER: 4.8 g PROTEIN: 1.1 g

Microwave the berries for 15 seconds, then sprinkle with sugar and lemon to taste. If you're feeling extra adventurous, skip the lemon and try some balsamic vinegar instead—it's an incredible flavor pairing.

This is not the most nutritious menu item, but it sure beats eating a bag of candy when you get a craving for something sweet and sour.

31. *Chocolate Banana Mash*

1 banana, mashed
¼ cup semisweet chocolate chips

CALORIES: 395 TOTAL FAT: 15 g FIBER: 7 g PROTEIN: 4 g

Everyone knows how to make chocolate-covered fruit, but this is a warm surprise that tastes remarkably like cookie dough. Mash the banana and sprinkle the chocolate chips over the top. Microwave for 15 seconds and check to see if the chocolate is melting. Stir and replace in the microwave for 10 more seconds. A very decadent, very special treat!

. . .

IT'S BEEN MY PLEASURE to share with you the insights I've acquired over my years living independently at college. College has been such a wonderful time in my life, and I'm sure it will be for you, too. You're entering a brand-new phase in your life, and there will be plenty of opportunities to learn your own lessons and forge your own experiences. I hope your new wealth of knowledge about how to eat, exercise, take supplements, and relax will help you navigate smoothly through your time at school and the rest of your life. Remember that independence is all about choice: You can choose to live healthfully and happily.

So take care of yourself. Use your new adult independence to take responsibility for your health and your life now. This way, you can be of great service to others, and be a happier you. I'd love to hear from you along the way! Come share your story at www.dormroomdiet.com. Good luck!!

REFERENCES

p. 51, Calculating BMR: www.shapefit.com/basal-metabolic-rate.html.

p. 53, Harris-Benedict Formula: www.bmi-calculator.net/bmr-calculator/bmr-formula.php

p. 67, Diet and calcium-rich foods: *International Journal of Obesity and Related Metabolic Disorders*, September 16, 2003.

p. 68, Teen soda consumption: *Time*, June 7, 2004, p. 84.

p. 135, Alcohol-related deaths: www.usatoday.com/news/health/2004-10-07-bingeusat_x.htm.

p. 145, Calories burned during exercise: www.nicotinefreekids.com/Frames/Pages/Exercise.html.

p. 177, Vitamin Supplements: Balch, James, and Mark Stengler. *Prescriptions for Natural Cures*. New York: Wiley, 2004.

p. 190, NHANES and B_6: *Well Being Journal*, March/April 2006.

p. 194, Dietary sources of vitamins: Carper, Jean. *Food: Your Miracle Medicine*. New York: HarperPerennial, 1994.

p. 212, Physical effects of stress: Sharma, Vijai P. *How Stress Affects the Body*. www.mindpub.com/art384.htm.

p. 219, Aromatherapy: Hirsch, Alan. *Scentsational Sex: The Secret to Using Aroma for Arousal*. Boston: Element Books, 1998.

REFERENCES

The following books were used as general reference guides.

Bottom Line Editors. *Uncommon Cures for Everyday Ailments.* Stamford, CT: Roundtable Press, 2005.

Goldberg, Donald P., Arnold Gitomer, and Robert Abel, Jr. *The Best Supplement for Your Health.* New York: Kensington, 2002.

Lemole, Gerald M. *The Healing Diet: A Total Health Program to Purify Your Lymph System and Reduce the Risk of Heart Disease and Cancer.* New York: HarperCollins, 2001.

Lieberman, Shari, and Nancy Bruning. *The Real Vitamin & Mineral Book: A Definitive Guide to Designing Your Personal Supplement Program.* New York: Penguin, 1997.

Murray, Michael, Joseph Pizzorno, and Lara Pizzorno. *The Encyclopedia of Healing Foods.* New York: Atria Books, 2005.

Documentary Films on Related Information:

Food, Inc. (2009)
King Corn (2007)
The Future of Food (2004)

Further Related Information on the Internet:

http://realfoodchallenge.org/

http://www.edibleschoolyard.org/

http://www.sfalliance.org/FSCbackground.html

http://www.bc.edu/clubs/realfood/realfoodnow.html

http://www.yale.edu/sustainablefood/farm.html

Further Reading:

What to Eat by Marion Nestle
Eating Animals by Jonathan Safran Foer
The Face on Your Plate: The Truth About Food by Jeffrey Moussaieff Masson
The Food Revolution by John Robbins and Dean Ornish
Diet for a Small Planet by Frances Moore Lappé
The China Study by T. Colin Campbell
Fast Food Nation by Eric Schlosser

INDEX

A

abdominal exercises, 168–73
addictive foods, 128–30
agave nectar, 97, 99
ailments and natural remedies
    cold remedies, 196–97
    constipation, 205–6
    diarrhea, 206–7
    fatigue, 202–3
    headache, 201
    insomnia, 203–4
    nausea and stomachache,
        198–99
    PMS and cramps, 199–201
    sore muscles and minor
        sprains, 202
    sore throat remedies,
        197–98
    urinary tract infection
        (UTI), 204
    yeast infection or vaginitis,
        204–5
alcoholic beverages, 78, 133,
    135, 136, 200
    binge drinking, 133, 135
    dangers of, 133, 135
almonds, 115–16
amino acids, 69

anemia, 180, 203
anorexia, 39, 40
antioxidants, 178, 186
apples, 65, 115–16
arnica, 202
aromatherapy, 219–23
artificial sweeteners, 64–65
asparagus and green bean tofu
    stir-fry, 273–74
athletic activity
        exercise (*See* exercise)
        weight, challenges of, 18
Atkins diet plan, 59
autonomy. *See* control of eating
avocado salad, 265–66
Ayoob, Keith-Thomas, 34

B

back exercises, 164–65
bad habits. *See* unhealthy
    eating
banana nut oatmeal, 257–58
Basal Metabolic Rate (BMR),
    50–54
        calculation of, 53–54
        factors affecting, 51–53
beans, 70, 271, 275–76
bedtime

eating before, 32
berries, 278
beverages
    alcoholic beverages, 78, 133,
        135, 136, 200
    artificial sweeteners, 64–65
    carbonation, 64
    fruit juices, 64
    sodas, 64–65, 66
    water, 31, 82
black bean, chickpea, lentil
    burgers, 275–76
blender recipes, 99, 101
body image, 38–39, 40
    taking stock, 48–50
    weight chart for women, 49
breakfast, 82, 256–57
breakfast recipes
    banana almond smoothie,
        261
    banana nut oatmeal, 257–58
    Greek yogurt with honey and
        chopped walnuts, 259–60
    nuttier butter, 257
    parfait, 260–61
    sandwiches, 258–59
    superfood breakfast
        smoothie, 262

breathing exercises, 213–16
bromelain, 202
brown rice with vegetables, 270–71
Brussels sprout chips, 271–72
bulimia, 39, 40
    case history, 43–47
butter, 67–68

C

cafeteria food
    farm-to-school program, 248, 249
    good and bad of, 95–99
    staff consultation, 249
caffeine, 200, 203
calcium, 64, 67–68, 204
    calcium-rich foods, 189
calorie counting, 74–75
carbohydrates. *See also* complex carbohydrates
    bread before meals, 81, 103
    daily portions, 73, 74
    grab-and-go foods, 75–77
    late-night simple carb loading, 117
    low-carb diets, 59–60
    pasta, 101–2, 103
    role of, 58–59
    simple and complex, 61–63, 72
    sources of, 59, 63–65
    tortilla wraps, in, 89
carbonation, 64
cardio workouts, 147–49
carrots, 70, 115–16
Celestial Seasonings
    Sleepytime tea, 204
    Throat Soothers tea, 198
    Tummy Mint tea, 198
certified humane livestocck, 244–45
cheese, 70
chest and triceps exercises, 155–59
chicken soup, 198

chili (vegetarian), 271
chocolate, 80–81, 115–16
    chocolate banana mash, 278
    strawberries dipped in, 99–100, 101
cod liver oil, 71, 187
coenzyme Q10, 201
coffee, 79–80
cold remedies, 196–97
college students
    all-nighters, 114–18
    cafeteria pros and cons, 95–99
    choices of food available, 87–89
    cooking for yourself, 253–56 (*See also* recipes)
    emotional eating and, 41–42
    family eating habits, effects of, 28–31
    freshmen weight gain, 27–28
    late-night talks, 126–28
    parties and campus gatherings, 121–23
    pressures on, 36–38, 211–13 (*See also* stress)
    price of food, effects of, 33–34, 91–93
    roommates, 37
    tailgating and sports events, 118–20
    time management, 90–91
complex carbohydrates
    baked goods, 76
    cereals, 75–76
    contrasted to simple, 62–63
    daily portions, 73, 74
    grab-and-go foods, 75–77
compote (fruit), 278
consciousness
    change of, 22–24
    consumer action for change, 246–50
    food choices, 229–30, 233–35, 240–50
    planetary health, 235–36

constipation remedies, 205–6
control of eating, 29, 30, 31
cost factors, 32–34, 91–93
    expense of good food, 230–33
cranberry, 204

D

dairy foods, 67–68
    butter, 67–68
    calcium in, 67, 68
    cheese, 70
    daily portions, 73, 74
    fat in, 67–68, 256
    vitamin D in, 67, 68
    yogurt, 65, 67, 99, 101, 259–60
dates (stuffed), 277
diarrhea remedies, 206–7
diet. *See* nutrition
Dietary Supplement Health and Education Act (DSHEA), 181
dieting
    fad diets, 5–6
    failures in, 57–61
    healthy lifestyle, 6–9
    negative aspects of, 5–6
    personal story, 8–11
    yo-yo dieting, 40
dinner, 270
dinner recipes
    black bean, chickpea, lentil burgers, 275–76
    brown rice with vegetables, 270–71
    Brussels sprout chips, 271–72
    candied sweet potato, 276
    quinoa with veggies, 272–73
    roasted vegetables, 274–75
    three bean vegetarian chili, 271
    tofu stir-fry with asparagus and green beans, 273–74
dormitory food, 99–101
dried fruits, 63, 77

E

eating disorders, 38–40
  anorexia, 39, 40
  Basal Metabolic Rate
    (BMR), effect on, 52
  body image and, 38–39
  bulimia, 39, 40, 43–47
echinacea, 197
eggs, 70
elderberry extract, 197
Emergen-C packets, 116
emotional eating, 6, 8, 40–42
  case history, 43–47
  defining, 40
  eating disorders, 40–42
  eradication of, 41–42,
    47–48
  warning signs, 42
  yo-yo dieting, 40
essential fatty acids (EFAs),
  70–72, 186
essential oils, 219–23
exercise, 35, 50, 139–40
  abdominals, 168–73
  back, 164–65
  balanced with food
    consumption, 73
  Basal Metabolic Rate (BMR)
    and, 52, 54
  cardio workouts, 147–49
  chest and triceps, 155–59
  cramps, PMS and, 200
  dorm room workout, 154–74
  endorphin release, 129
  excuses for avoiding, 142–45
  getting food yourself, 98
  goal, setting of, 143–44
  importance of, 140–42
  lack of, 34–35
  legs, 159–64
  lengthening and
    strengthening workouts,
    151–53
  Pilates, 151, 153
  plan, creation of, 146–47
  sample workout, 154–74

shoulders and biceps,
  165–68
sore muscles and minor
  sprains, remedies for, 202
specific muscle group
  training, 149–51
stopping and starting again,
  147
stretching, 153–54
target heart rate (THR),
  148–49
time factors, 144–45
TV watching, with, 123
variation, importance of,
  146–47, 150–51
walking, 132
warm-up, 155
yoga, 151–53

F

faith and meaning, 223–25
family eating habits, 28–31
farming. *See also* food supply
  farmer's market, 250
  industrial and traditional,
    236–41
  locally-produced foods,
    245–46
Fast Food Nation (Schlosser),
  106
fast food tips, 104–6
fatigue remedies, 202–3
fats
  daily portions, 73, 74
  dairy products, 67–68
  essential fatty acids (EFAs),
    70–72, 186
  good fats, 70–72
  hydrogenated fats, 256
  "low fat" deceptions, 97
  omega 3 fats, 71–72, 201
fear of success, 15–16
fiber, 62–63, 72–73
fish, 70, 71
folic acid, foods high in,
  190–91

food supply
  certified humane livestock,
    244–45
  consumer action for change,
    246–50
  farm-to-school program,
    248, 249
  free-range and grass-fed,
    244
  government policies, 33
  industrial agriculture, 236–
    38, 239, 240–41
  locally-produced foods,
    245–46
  organic food, 241–44
  price of good food, 32–34,
    230–33
  Standard American Diet
    (SAD), 32–34
  subsidies for certain foods,
    231–33
  traditional *vs.* industrial
    farms, 238–39
free-range animals, 244
fried foods, 98, 103, 104, 105
fruits and vegetables, 63–65,
  70
  dried fruits, 63, 77
  good choices, 64, 77
  juices, 64
  before meals, 103
  recipes (*See* recipes)
  washing before eating, 255

G

games, 130–31, 132
garlic greens, 268–69
Gatorade, 198–99
gazpacho, 264–65
ghrelin hormone, 66
glucagon, 72
glucose levels, 59
goals
  exercise goals, 143–44
  first short-term goal, 24
grapefruit, 115–16

grass-fed animals, 244
grocery shopping, 93
gycogen levels, 59–60

H
hands, activities for, 130–32
Harper, Joel, 154
headache remedies, 201
health food, 93
healthy eating
    age countdown, 83, 112
    balance, importance of, 73,
        96, 99
    cafeteria food, good and bad
        of, 95–99
    conscious choices, 233–35
    cooking for yourself, 253–56
        (See also recipes)
    cost factors, 32–34, 91–93,
        230–33
    fast food tips, 104–6
    five principles of, 82–84
    frequency of eating, 83
    grab-and-go foods, 75–77
    half portions, 98
    indulgences, 110–13
    late night studying, 115–18
    late-night talks, 127–28
    moderation, 110–13, 119,
        120, 129–30
    parties and campus
        gatherings, 122–23
    planetary health and,
        235–36
    restaurants, in, 101–3
    storage space for food,
        93–94
    tailgating and sports events,
        120
    time factors, 90–91
    TV watching, during,
        125–26
heat as remedy, 201
high-fructose corn syrup, 230,
    256

I
immune system
    stress, effects of, 212–13
    vitamins and, 181, 182–84
industrial agriculture, 236–38,
    239, 240–41
insomnia remedies, 203–4
insulin, 62, 72, 99–100
irradiated foods, 242

J
junk food, 17–19
    price and policy, 32–34

K
Kabat-Zinn, Jon, 217
kale chips, 263–64
kale salad, 264
knitting, 131

L
late-night talks, 126–28
leg exercises, 159–64
legumes, 70
lengthening and strengthening
    workouts, 151–53
lentil burgers, 275–76
lentil salad, 266–67
local foods, 245–46
lunch, 262–63
lunch recipes and dishes
    crunchy avocado salad,
        265–66
    garlic greens, 268–69
    gazpacho, 264–65
    kale chips, 263–64
    kale salad, 264
    lentil salad, 266–67
    miso soup, 263
    spinach soup, 269
    vegan tofu dog sandwich,
        266
    vinaigrettes, 267–68

M
magnesium, 199–200, 201, 204

margarine, 67–68
massage and reflexology, 218
mealtime
    bread before meals, 81, 103
    breakfast, importance of, 82
    college communal dining,
        37–38
    family eating habits, 29–31
    fruit before meals, 103
    glass of water before, 31, 82
    preparation of meals, 29, 31
    recipes for breakfast, lunch,
        and dinner (See specific
        subject headings)
    two hours before bed, 32, 83
meat. See protein
meditation, 216–17
menstruation, 180
Metamucil, 72, 205, 206
mineral supplements. See
    vitamins and supplements
miso soup, 198, 263
mononucleosis, 203
myrrh, 197

N
nausea and stomacheache
    remedies, 198–99
NutriBiotic's Grapefruit Seed
    Extract, 198
nutrition, 49–50
    awareness of, 30, 31
    Basal Metabolic Rate
        (BMR), effect on, 52–53
    calorie counting, 74–75
    carbohydrate facts, 58–63
    conscious food choices,
        229–30, 233–35, 240–50
        (See also consciousness;
        food supply)
    daily portions, 73–74
    dairy foods, 67–68
    fiber, importance of, 62–63,
        72–73
    foods high in nutrients,
        189–95

food supply issues (*See* food supply)

fruits and vegetables, 63–65

price of good food, 32–34, 230–33

protein, 68–70

vitamins and supplements (*See* vitamins and supplements)

O

obesity, rise in, 34–35

olive oil, 71, 81, 103

omega 3 fats, 71–72, 201

organic food, 241–44

osteoporosis, 64, 68, 179, 185

overeating, 17–19

artificial sweeteners and, 65

ghrelin signals, 66

portions, importance of, 73–74

P

parfait, 260–61

pasta, 101–2, 103

peanut butter, 65, 70

pears, 115–16

peer pressure, 36–38

personal story

adolescence, 17–21

consciousness change, 22–24

dieting, 8–11

overeating, 17–19

research on eating, 20–21

size in childhood, 16–18

Pilates exercise, 151, 153

PMS and cramps, remedies for, 199–201

pollution and vitamins, 181

polypeptides, 69

portions, importance of, 73–74

potassium-rich foods, 191–92

potato chips, 63

poultry, 70

Price, Weston, 180–81

price of food, 32–34, 230–33

probiotics, 205, 207

processed foods, 32–34, 180

protein, 68–70

daily portions, 73, 74

good and bad types of, 68–70

red meat consumption, 73, 74

too much, effects of, 69

Q

questions to post, 24

quinoa with veggies, 272–73

R

radishes, 65

RealAge.com, 182

recipes. *See also* specific meals and dishes

basic guidelines, 255–56

breakfast, 256–62

dinner, 270–76

levels of difficulty, 254–55

lunch, 262–69

snacks, 277–78

religious practice, 223–24

remedies for ailments. *See* ailments and natural remedies

restaurants, 101–3

fast food, 104–6

roasted vegetables, 274–75

roommates, 37

S

salads

avocado salad, 265–66

kale salad, 264

lentil salad, 266–67

vinaigrettes, 267–68

sandwiches

breakfast sandwiches, 258–59

vegan tofu dog sandwich, 266

Schlosser, Eric, 106

sedentary lifestyles, 34–35

selenium-rich foods, 192

serotonin levels, 60

shoulders and biceps exercises, 165–68

skin probelms, 179

sleep, 200

smoking, 133–35, 136, 200

smoothies, 261, 262

snacks, 29

chocolate banana mash, 278

fruit compote, 278

good choices, 65

grab-and-go foods, 75–77

healthy late-night snacks, 115–16

stuffed dates, 277

TV watching, during, 123–26

sodas, 64–65, 66, 68

sodium, 97

sore muscle and sprain remedies, 202

sore throat remedies, 197–98

soup, 198

gazpacho, 264–65

miso soup, 263

spinach soup, 269

spices and herbs, 256

spinach soup, 269

sports events, 118–20

Standard American Diet (SAD), 32–34, 180–81

stir-fry recipe, 273–74

storage space for food, 93–94

stress, 36–38, 114–18

aromatherapy for coping, 219–23

breathing exercise for coping, 213–16

faith and meaning, 223–25

fight or flight, effects of, 212–13

massage and reflexology for coping, 218

INDEX

stress (*continued*)
    meditation for coping,
      216–17
stretching, importance of,
    153–54
studying/writing papers,
    114–18
subsidies in agriculture, 231–33
success
    fear of, 15–16
    past, building on, 24
sweet potato (candied), 276

T

tailgating and sports events,
    118–20
target heart rate (THR),
    148–49
tea, 198, 201, 204
three bean vegetarian chili, 271
Time magazine, 68
time management, 90–91
    exercise, time for, 144–45
tofu, 70, 266, 273–74
tortilla wraps, 89
Traditional Medicinals
    PMS tea, 201
    Throat Coat, 198
transformative questions,
    23–24
TV watching, 123–26

U

unhealthy eating, 17–19
    addictive foods, 128–30
    alternative activities for your
      hands, 130–32
    college pressures causing,
      36–38
    distracted eating, 29, 30, 32,
      109–10
    family eating habits, 29–31
    late-night simple carb
      loading, 117
    late-night talks, 126–27
    list of temptations, 78

"low fat" deceptions, 97
parties, etc, 121–22
price of food, 32–34
Standard American Diet
    (SAD), 32–34, 180–81
studying for tests, 114, 117
tailgating and sports events,
    118–20
TV watching, during,
    123–25
writing papers, 114, 117
urinary tract infection (UTI)
    remedies, 204

V

vaginitis remedies, 204–5
vegetarian chili, 271
vinaigrette recipes, 267–68
vitamins and supplements
    ailments and remedies
      using, 195–207 (*See also*
      ailments and natural
      remedies)
    antioxidants, 178, 186
    B and food sources, 190–91,
      199
    basic supplement plan,
      186–87
    C and food sources, 193–94,
      196
    choosing supplements, 185
    cold remedies, 196–97
    cost factors, 184–85
    D from foods, sun, or
      supplement, 67, 68, 187,
      196
    E and food sources, 195
    Emergen-C packets, 116
    essential fatty acids (EFAs),
      186
    foods high in vitamins and
      minerals, 189–95
    immune system and, 181,
      182–84
    liquid vitamin drinks, 189
    minerals, 186

multivitamins, 186
pollution effects, defense
    against, 181
reasons for supplements,
    179–81
recommended daily
    allowance chart, 188
safety of supplements, 182
sore throat remedies,
    197–98
supplements explained,
    178–79
treatment of sicknesses, 181

W

walnuts, 257, 259, 260, 277
water
    daily consumption, 82
    glass or two before meals, 31
weight chart, 49
weight loss
    fiber, effects of, 72–73
    low-fat dairy products and,
      67
    omega fats, role of, 71–72
Weleda Ratanhia Mouthwash,
    197
*Wherever You Go, There You
Are* (Kabat-Zinn), 217
whole grains, 61–63, 70
    fiber source, 62–63, 72

Y

yeast infection remedies,
    204–5
yoga, 151–53
yogurt, 65, 67
    blender recipes, 99, 101
    Greek yogurt with honey and
      chopped walnuts, 259–60
yo-yo dieting, 40

Z

zinc and food sources, 192–93,
    197

ABOUT THE AUTHOR

DAPHNE OZ is a 2008 graduate of Princeton University, and the author of the national bestseller *The Dorm Room Diet*, first published in 2006. Daphne and her book have been featured in *The New York Times, People, Reader's Digest, Teen Vogue, Seventeen, Cosmo Girl!,* and *The Wall Street Journal,* and on *Good Morning America, The Tyra Banks Show, Fox & Friends,* and *NPR Weekend Edition.*

Daphne is developing a campaign to raise youth awareness about health access and food politics in America, combining web, television, and print platforms. She is an in-demand speaker on health, diet, and wellness issues facing teens and young adults.

The daughter of Dr. Mehmet Oz and Lisa Oz, co-authors of the #1 *New York Times* bestselling *You* books, Daphne grew up in Cliffside Park, New Jersey, and now resides in New York City.

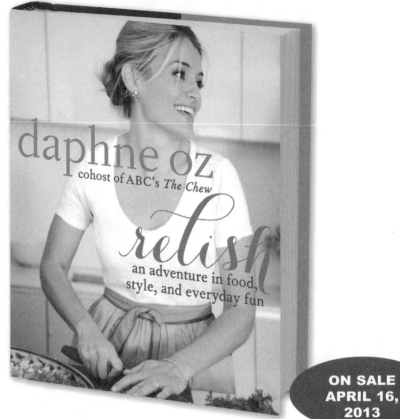
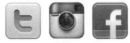